Blepharoplasty

Everything You Need to Know about Revitalizing Your Aging Eyes

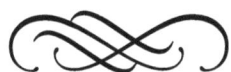

Dr. Edwin Williams

ISBN-10: 1518721796
ISBN-13: 9781518721793
Library of Congress Control Number: 2015918825
CreateSpace Independent Publishing Platform
North Charleston, South Carolina

Additional Books by Dr. Edwin Williams

Rhinoplasty: Everything You Need to Know about Fixing and Reshaping Your Nose

While there are many blepharoplasty surgeons who have mentored me and taught me the principles of blepharoplasty, it is my patients who have been my greatest teachers. They have given me countless opportunities to develop as a surgeon and as a person, teaching me some of life's most valuable lessons in the process.

It is with appreciation and gratitude that I dedicate this book to them.

Special Thanks

A special thank you to the very talented people, especially the staff of the Williams Center for Plastic Surgery, who contributed to this project, including

Susan Sullivan, RN, chief operating officer for the Williams Center—for her constant insight, guidance, and support;

Merci Miglino, editor and writer—for her guidance and creative influence; and my wife, Cherie, and our children, Katie, Riley, Lydia, and Evan—for their constant support and understanding, which has allowed me to achieve this next level in my surgical career.

Table of Contents

Intro

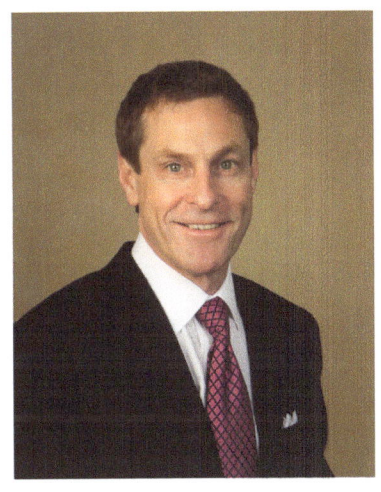

The art of facial surgery is bringing the face into balance without losing the unique characteristics that define the patient's identity. My intent in writing this book is to answer your questions about blepharoplasty, or eyelid surgery and let you in on what I, as an experienced board-certified facial plastic surgeon, have learned over the years.

As we age, the excess skin and fatty accumulation often make the opening of the eyes look tired, dull, or even sinister. After performing this complex yet common procedure some several thousand times, I have become especially tuned-in to what patients want to know before making the decision to proceed with blepharoplasty. The very first thing I do in my consultations, before I even share the specifics about what I see, is ask what you don't like about your eyes. I listen to what is said (and not said). If you say, "I look tired," that might mean one thing to you and another to me as a surgeon, so listening with the intent to really understand your concerns is essential if I am to help set and meet your expectations.

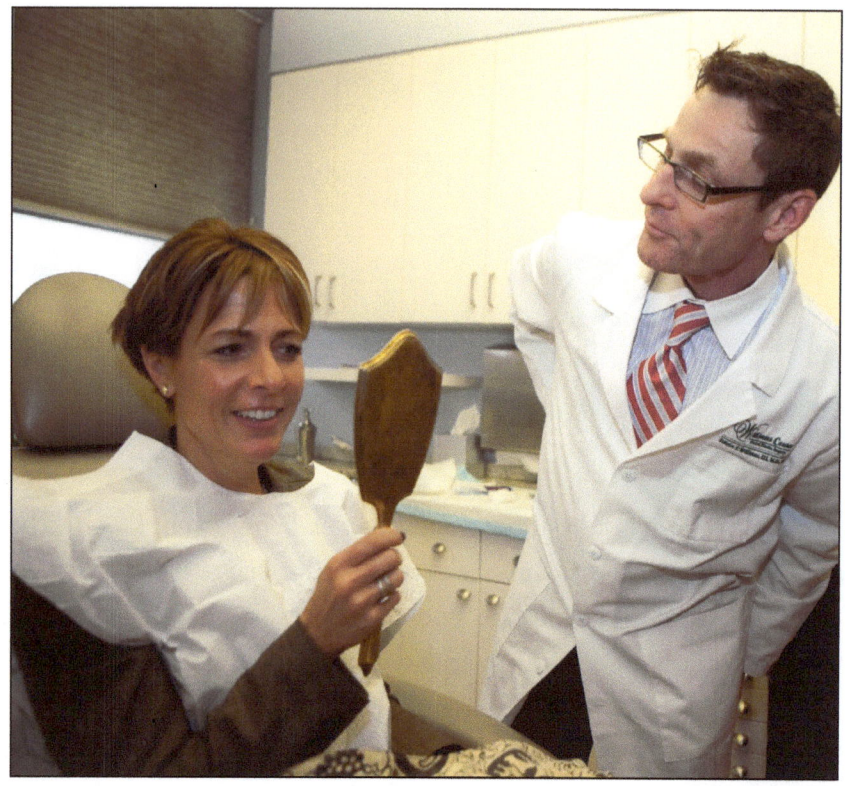

Patients may not be able to articulate their concerns. That's when I say, "Well, let me tell you what I see. I'm going to use some medical terms, but then I'm going to try to communicate it in a way that you can relate to." As I observe your eyes and share what I see, I might talk about *ptosis*, for example, which simply means your upper lids droop and cover the pupils.

If I don't take the opportunity to *really* listen to you, I could miss an essential aspect of what changes are important to you. I understand that for many patients it's difficult to speak up when they perceive someone's expertise as beyond theirs. However, I encourage you to make every effort to share what you want and don't want. Give your surgeon every opportunity to meet your expectations and needs with his or her expertise and skill—the result of which is something both of you can feel great about.

Real-Life Aging Process

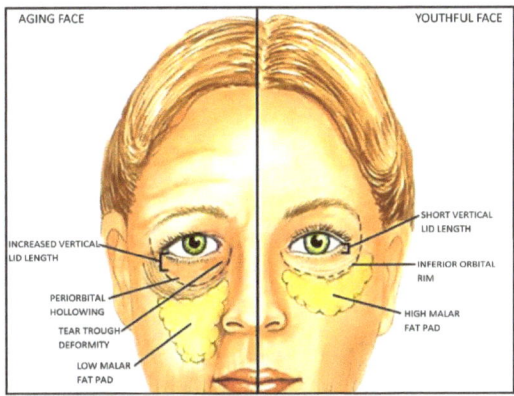

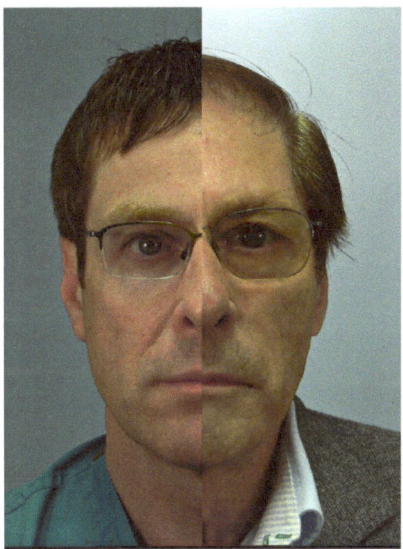

This is a split-face photograph of me on the left and my father on the right. I find this an interesting study of the aging process and have done this same comparison with mother/daughter photographs.

As you can see from this photo and graphic, the aging process is not simply about wrinkles and bulging or puffy lower lids. The process results in deflation, loss of tissue elasticity, and a more elongated distance between the lower lid and the top of the cheek.

ABOUT THOSE SMILE LINES

"Wrinkles should merely indicate where the smiles have been." —Mark Twain

Smile lines often bother my patients, and, unfortunately, there are limited ways to treat those crinkly areas around the lines that can extend into the midface area. While blepharoplasty cannot address crow's-feet, it can remove some of the excess skin and a small amount of the wrinkling.

As Mark Twain wisely notes, these lines are caused by smiling and other regular facial expressions. It is the underlying muscle that causes that wrinkling, so the only way to successfully treat it is with Botox or an aggressive skin resurfacing, whether it's a chemical peel or laser resurfacing.

Chapter 1

The Eyes: The Window to the Refreshed Soul

The Anatomy of the Eye

Let's talk about the anatomy of the eye as it relates to eye-lifts, or blepharoplasty. The eye is a very complex structure, and you do not need to fully understand its many attributes to get a clear picture of what is involved in blepharoplasty. I've included this rather medical explanation to better inform you of what blepharoplasty does and does not include and to offer assurance that the chance of vision changes is extraordinarily low.

Always make sure you are working with a well-qualified, board-certified surgeon with a considerable amount of experience with eyelid surgery. It is important to note that not all board-certified surgeons are experienced in eyelid surgery.

The eyelids serve multiple purposes, including protecting the eyeball from injury, controlling the amount of light that enters the eye, and lubricating the eyeball with tears secreted by the lacrimal gland during blinking. Together, these functions help maintain the structural integrity of the eyeball and protect it from damage.

The eyelid consists primarily of skin, underlying soft tissue, also called subcutaneous tissue, and a thin layer of muscle called the *orbicularis oculi*. Under this muscle are other tissues that divide the area into different planes. Also, there are lid retractors that allow the eyelids to open and assist in blinking.

The levator muscle and the eyelid margin are responsible for opening the upper eyelid. With age the muscle can become dysfunctional and droop, which results in *ptosis*.

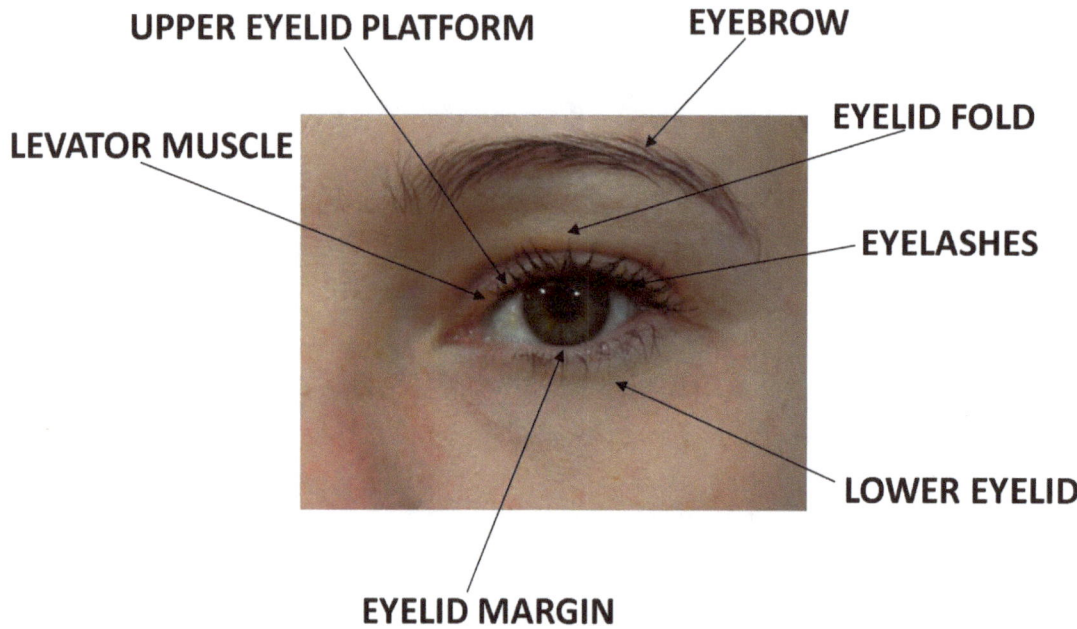

Chapter 2

Why Consider Blepharoplasty?

According to the American Society of Plastic Surgeons, over two hundred thousand people a year in the United States choose cosmetic eyelid surgery. Since you are reading this book, I'm going to assume you are considering such surgery (*blepharoplasty*). You may be noticing that you look tired and stressed even when you are well-rested. You may have droopy upper lids that are affecting your vision or have bulging or hollowness that seems to be getting progressively more pronounced as you age.

Perhaps a friend has had a blepharoplasty or brow lift and you notice how much happier your friend is with his or her new appearance and how your friend feels about himself or herself as a result. Or maybe you always wanted to explore what the surgical versus nonsurgical options can do to enhance your looks or create a younger-looking and more vital appearance. Whatever the reason, you want to know exactly what to expect from a blepharoplasty.

First, let me say that the ideal goal for any plastic surgery is to improve the face aesthetically, making sure it harmonizes with other facial features for a more natural, normal appearance. To give my patients the best opportunity to visualize what's possible for their unique features and to determine whether their expectations are realistic, I use a computerized imager during the initial consultation.

A CGI is Worth a Thousand Words

You may be reluctant to have a blepharoplasty because you're afraid your eyes will not be what you expected or wanted. Computer-generated imagery (CGI) can help alleviate such fears as it gives you and your surgeon a visual idea of the goals for the surgery.

That's why computer imaging is an essential part of my practice: it allows patients to communicate their aesthetic wishes in visual form. At the same time, it gives me the opportunity to display what sort of results I feel are achievable and realistic given the patient's facial anatomy and skin type. There is no guarantee your eyes will look exactly like the ones shown to you in the simulation, but it can help you feel more confident in proceeding with surgery.

How Exactly Does CGI Work?

At the time of your visit, photos are taken and put on the *imager*, a computer with a screen for viewing. These images usually take about fifteen to twenty minutes to create. The images are not a guarantee of results but rather a visual representation of our mutual surgical goals for your blepharoplasty or brow lift.

In each case, we recognize that everyone's eyes are different and surgery should be tailored to match one's anatomy and other facial features. A "cookie cutter" approach may result in an artificial appearance for some patients.

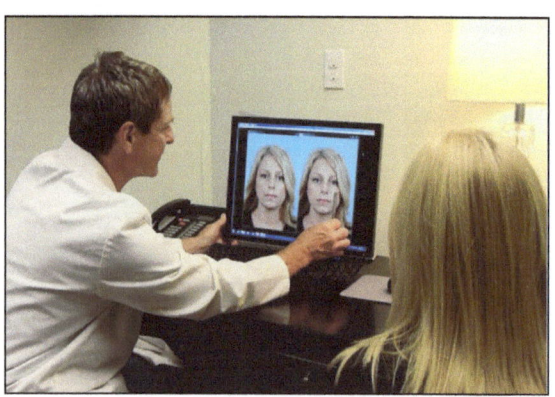

Computer-generated imagery (CGI) is a specialized application of computer graphics that allows me to manipulate a photograph and explain and develop possible surgical goals, and do so right before the patient's eyes. This is extremely helpful in effective communication between doctor and patient. The goals of one patient may be very different from another. One of the integral parts of my practice is making sure each procedure is a fully unique event. I am not creating the same "look" for everyone; I am partnering with my patient to create a customized surgical plan that honors his or her unique characteristics, including ethnicity.

Ideal Candidates for Upper and Lower Blepharoplasty and Brow Lifts

Good candidates for blepharoplasty and brow lifts include men and women who are physically healthy; realistic in their expectations; and looking to improve the appearance of puffy under-eye bags, circles, drooping, or wrinkles in the eyelid area.

The people who get the most from this procedure are those who live a healthy lifestyle—avoiding smoking, insomnia, sun exposure, and other stressors.

Although most patients are between forty and sixty, nonsurgical techniques as well as blepharoplasty and brow lifts may be performed at any age when the face and forehead area have begun to show the signs of aging. At our center, each patient is carefully evaluated to determine the best approach for his or her goals.

Watch a Real Life Blepharoplasty Consultation with Computer Imaging

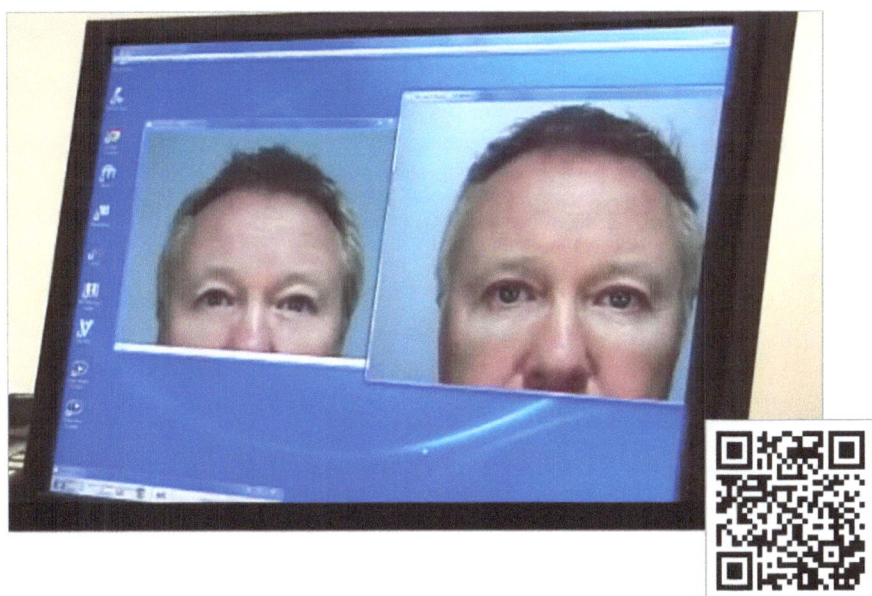

Ethnicity and Anatomy Differences

There are a number of anatomic differences between an Asian patient's upper eyelid, which does not have a fold, and that of a Caucasian patient. At least 50 percent of Asians have a single eyelid, which is to say that the eyelid has no crease and more fat tissue. The skin fold, covering the inner corner periorbital fat (the tissues surrounding or lining the orbit of the eye pads), contributes to the "puffiness" and further obscures the crease. Also, the levator muscle, which adheres to the fascia and attaches to the skin, tends to be weak or nonexistent, and the fat pad in the upper and lower lids tends to be thicker.

Another anatomical difference in the upper eyelids of Asians is the presence of an epicanthal fold—the skin fold of the upper eyelid covering the inner angle of the eye—which obscures the inner corner of the eye and gives it a relatively narrow appearance.

As we enter our forties, fifties, and beyond, the tired look of the eyelids continues to advance. Often, the lower-eyelid muscle loosens and falls, further accentuating the appearance of fatigue. In the following chapters, we take a look at each of these options as well cosmetic alternatives, such as Botox, Restylane, Juvéderm, and other injectables, that *temporarily* address eye wrinkles and lines.

Chapter 3

Blepharoplasty and Brow-Lift Procedures

Let me correct a common misconception with the term "eyelid lift," which is often used interchangeably with blepharoplasty. The eyelid is not actually lifted during blepharoplasty surgery. Instead, a blepharoplasty removes excess skin, muscle, and sometimes fat from the upper or lower eyelids. In some cases you might need only skin removed, but not muscle, or you might need the procedure done on both upper and lower eyelids.

An upper or lower eyelid surgery includes the midface, from the medial *canthus* to the lateral *canthus*—that is, from the upper part of the lower eyelid down to the corner of the mouth. The eyelid does not stop at the shadow area; it's considered one contiguous piece of anatomy.

As a surgeon I can improve your appearance and functional problems with your eyelids by rejuvenating the area surrounding your eyes.

Blepharoplasty (both upper and lower) specifically addresses the following conditions:

- Excess fatty deposits that appear as puffiness in the upper eyelids, typically in the corners
- Loose or sagging skin that creates folds or disturbs the natural contour of the upper eyelid, sometimes impairing vision

- Excess skin and fine wrinkles of the lower eyelid
- Bags under the eyes
- Hollowness and circles
- Droopiness of the lower eyelids, showing white below the iris (color portion of the eye), due to loose muscle (ptosis)
- Droopiness of the upper eyelids due to laxity in the muscle (ptosis)

In addition, a brow-lift procedure, also known as a forehead lift or upper facelift, can minimize the signs of aging in the forehead. As we get older, our eyebrows can appear heavy and contribute to an aged appearance of the upper eyes and eyelid complex. If the eyebrows have descended so they appear too low or are pushing down on what we call the orbital bones, then a brow lift may prove to be beneficial.

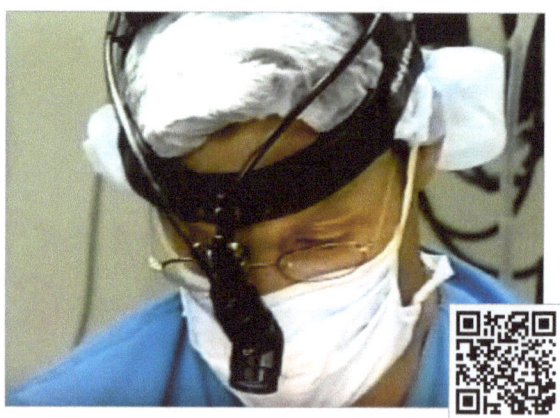

Upper-Eyelid Surgery

Droopy eyelids are a major reason people consider upper-eyelid blepharoplasty, which removes and tightens excess eyelid skin for a more alert and youthful appearance.

The Sliver Technique

At our center we perform what we call the "sliver technique" on the upper eyelids to remove loose, excess skin. A fine incision is made in the upper eyelid's crease or just under the eyelashes for a lower-eyelid *sliver*. A small amount of excess skin is removed and sewn together with a very fine suture. The sutures are removed in about six days.

The "sliver" blepharoplasty surgery alone can be performed under local anesthesia with or without oral sedation in a surgeon's office. As long as the patient does not request oral sedation, the patient is able to drive himself or herself home.

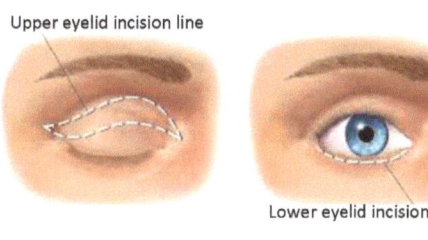

Upper eyelid incision line

Lower eyelid incision line

Blepharoplasty

Eyelid Ptosis

Drooping of the upper eyelids is referred to as *ptosis* and usually occurs when the muscle of the upper eyelid is not strong enough to raise the eyelids, resulting in the eyelids resting over part of the iris (colored part of eye). Here, the muscle is surgically tightened in the upper eyelid.

While *mild ptosis* repair is considered a cosmetic procedure, *severe ptosis* is considered a functional blepharoplasty performed for medical reasons. If the eyelid droops low enough to impair your vision, your procedure could be covered by insurance, which requires a field-of-vision study. This study is performed in your eye doctor's office and is a quick, easy test.

Lower-Eyelid Surgery

Lower blepharoplasty removes excess skin and bulging fat and reduces wrinkles to improve the shape of the lower eyelid. Sometimes tightening the eyelid is needed to correct droopiness or sagging. Adding fat is done to improve a "hollowed" appearance to the eye area, which can also help to smooth the skin.

Lower-eyelid surgery often involves skin incisions directly below the lash line or on the inside of the lower eyelid. When there is bulging fat, an inside incision is needed on the lower eyelid. This is considered a *transconjunctival approach*. This allows for access to the eyelid fat without visible incisions, making this technique perfect for patients who need fat removed. This approach can be combined with laser resurfacing or a chemical peel of the eyelid skin to reduce lines and wrinkles if removal of skin is not needed.

We believe that volumetric restoration using fat transfer is an integral part of lower-eyelid procedures in most patients. It not only rejuvenates the lower eyelid but also helps address the aging in the midface by softening the folds around the nose and mouth. A key point is treating the eyelid and midface together by using fat transfers.

Lower-eyelid surgery typically takes sixty to ninety minutes and may be performed in a surgeon's office-based facility, an outpatient surgery center, like our New England Laser and Cosmetic Surgery Center, or a hospital. We prefer to perform blepharoplasty with a combination of local anesthesia and IV sedation, or "twilight sleep." In the local mixture, there is a small concentration of epinephrine, which constricts blood vessels and helps reduce bleeding. You will not feel the injection of local anesthesia, as it is administered while you are already sedated. Blepharoplasty can be performed on upper eyelids or lower eyelids—or both at the same time.

Your surgeon might give you a choice regarding anesthesia, depending on your particular circumstances. If you have any concerns, don't hesitate to ask your surgeon why he or she is recommending a particular anesthesia.

Fat Transfer: The Facts

Often patients ask, "Why do you take fat out of the eye area and add it from another part of my body?" The simple answer is this: it's different fat. If you take the bulging fat around the eye out and just move it back in, it doesn't have the longevity of the fat we harvest from the abdomen or thigh, which is done with an incision that is approximately a half-inch long and requires one or two stitches.

The most common place we end up harvesting fat from is the abdomen, and a little bit of fat goes a long way. If we have someone who's very thin, we'll take it from the outer or inner thigh. However, by and large, we can almost always get enough from the abdomen. And studies show there's no one area that seems to be better than the abdomen as far as retention and longevity are concerned.

We harvest the fat under very low pressure, using a hand syringe as to not injure the fat cells. Then we spin the fat in a centrifuge and separate the broken cells from the viable cells. We take the viable fat cells and put them in very small syringes and slowly and precisely inject them in kind of a microdroplet (pearl technique) into these tiny tunnels close to the muscle and blood supply.

We follow the patient's own bone structure as the shape of the face stays the same. For example, if you have high cheekbones, you will continue to have them, but if you do not, you will not have them as a result of this procedure. Fat transfer is not about giving you a "fat" face; it's about restoring the fat lost during the aging process and replacing it in a naturally flattering way.

With fat transfer we do not want to overcorrect or overcompensate for the fat we lose as we age. We want results that are natural looking. This is a valuable enhancement to the procedure that we didn't have before. It lasts longer than any of the injectables, which are shorter term (about a year). I often tell my patients that we don't know exactly how long fat transfers last because we lose a small amount each year as our faces naturally age. The good news is we can always add a little more fat as there's basically an unlimited amount.

Weight Changes and Fat Transfer

If you gain a significant amount of weight after eyelid surgery with fat transfer, it will likely show up as more volume in the face. When you lose it, you can see that effect in the face as well.

Over the years, my patients have told me their skin looks better after having fat transfers to their faces. We now know this is not just anecdotal, but, in fact, the skin does have an improved appearance, likely due to growth factors from stem cells that are transferred within the fat. This change is usually visible six to twelve months after the procedure. When you look at the before and after photos in this book, you will notice the skin on these individuals does indeed appear younger.

Real Patient Experience

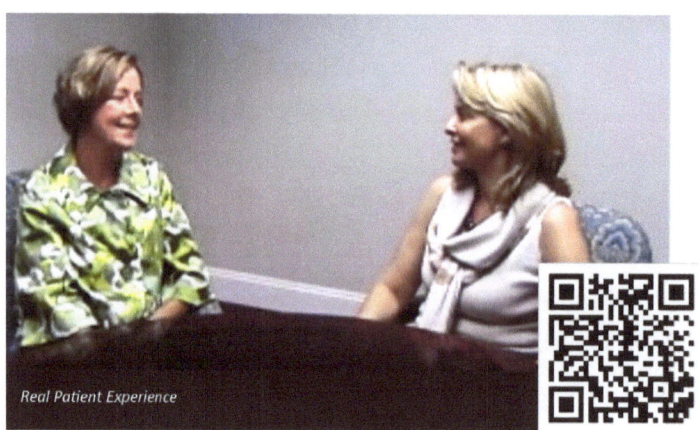

Real Patient Experience

Dr. Williams' patient talks about her upper eye lid repair and lower lid blepharoplasty with fat transfer.

Brow Lift/Forehead Lift

We usually recommend brow-lift surgery when the eyebrow is unnaturally low and there is a short distance between the eyebrows and lashes. Having a droopy brow line is often a sign of age, but it can also be hereditary. In some rare instances, people in their teens will develop eyebrow droop, making them appear older.

Brow and forehead lifts are designed to elevate and separate the eyebrows and reduce ridges and furrows on the forehead. Forehead lifts are done through mini-incisions using endoscopic tools. A well-done procedure avoids a "surprised" look and presents a natural opening up of the facial expression around the eyes.

At the Williams Center, we perform a unique version of the brow lift that lifts the midface as well. This procedure actually lifts two-thirds of the upper face and is done through the same incisions required in a brow lift alone. There are five small incisions made and hidden in the hairline so they are not noticeable even when the hair is worn up. These incisions are closed with surgical clips, not sutures, and present little risk of hair loss.

This procedure achieves an excellent correction of a drooping brow and requires less recovery time.

There is a misconception among patients that a brow lift will make their foreheads appear too large; however, when the procedure is done correctly, this is not the case at all. If you think about it, the distance from the eyebrow to the hairline is constant. Over time the tissue moves downward, crowding the visual field or lower part of the forehead. When this is moved up, the distance really is unchanged; however, the patient looks more bright-eyed and refreshed.

On rare occasions we will have a patient who has an extremely high forehead. In this case the brow lift performed is referred to as a *trichophytic brow lift*. Trichophytic closures involve overlapping the edges of the incision when suturing or stapling them. One side of the existing skin is cut at an oblique angle, after which the adjacent skin flaps are brought together to close the incision.

Rather than placing the incision behind the hairline, which would move the hairline back further and increase the height of the brow, we make the incision at the junction of the forehead and hairline. This shortens the forehead a bit (the distance from the eyebrow to the hairline) by moving the forehead up and only eliminating the skin at the highest aspect of the brow. The incision in this particular situation is very well hidden and acceptable to most individuals with a high hairline.

Brow-lift surgery may be performed in surgeon's office-based facilities, an outpatient surgery center, like our New England Laser and Cosmetic Surgery Center, or a hospital. The procedure typically takes one to two hours and can be performed with either local anesthesia with IV sedation or general anesthesia. You will not feel the injection of local anesthesia as it is administered while you are already sedated.

In the mixture, there is a small concentration of epinephrine, which constricts blood vessels and helps reduce bleeding.

Your surgeon may give you a choice regarding anesthesia, depending on your particular circumstances. If you have any concerns, don't hesitate to ask why a particular anesthesia is recommended.

After a brow lift, some swelling, bruising, and temporary numbness of the scalp may occur. Patients may experience some discomfort or a headache, and this can be controlled with pain medication. Itching may also occur. Head dressings will be removed within three days after surgery, and patients should keep the head elevated during this time. Surgical clips will be removed in one week, and this is typically painless.

Most of the swelling and bruising should fade within about a week or two. Endoscope procedures typically involve less bruising and swelling and a reduced recovery period. Patients are typically able to return to work in about seven to ten days. More strenuous activities will need to be postponed for several weeks, and sun exposure should be limited for several months.

As with all types of surgery, there are potential risks associated with brow lifts, and these may include the following: adverse anesthesia reactions, asymmetry, bleeding, infection, nerve injury, and the need for additional surgery. These potential complications are extraordinarily rare at the hands of an experienced surgeon.

Blepharoplasty or Brow Lift?

For patients with droopy upper eyes, this can be a complex issue. Typically, the excess skin that is hanging over the upper eyelid is addressed by an upper-eyelid blepharoplasty. This is usually sufficient for most patients.

The tissue that is hanging down upward of the eye and drooping or crowding the upper-eyelid field can extend from the brow toward the temple area, and to address that area typically involves a brow lift as seen in the before and after photos below:

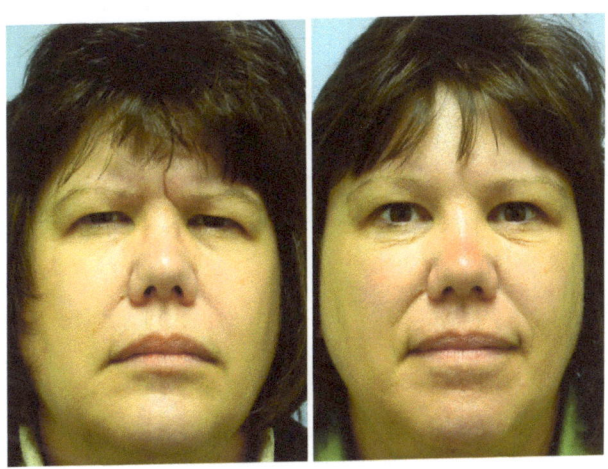

One way to decide whether a brow lift might be for you is to compare your eyebrows as they appear today against a series of photographs of yourself when you were younger. A picture truly is worth a thousand words when you are unsure which cosmetic surgical procedure will address your concerns.

Many patients with a heavy brow benefit from both a brow lift and an upper-eyelid blepharoplasty, and we typically include the upper eyelids at no additional charge to the patient. When someone has a heavy brow, we do not want to overdo the upper eyelid to compensate for the brow by removing too much skin from the eyelid. It is best to address each area accordingly.

Where to Have Your Blepharoplasty Surgery

I've chosen to operate in my own accredited ambulatory surgery center. I believe this is the optimal situation for my patients since I have all the essential backup systems and the same safety standards as a hospital. We have all the rigors and standards of a federally inspected hospital *without* any unnecessary exposure to germs and illnesses.

While a surgeon can also get his or her office accredited to accommodate an operating room, an accredited ambulatory surgery center operates at a much higher standard. In my center, for example, we have climate-controlled air exchanges that comply with hospital standards. In short our operating rooms are identical to those in a hospital; we're just not attached to one.

Also, the same team works with the patient throughout the surgical procedure and postoperative period, rather than sharing a recovery room with multiple patients, and our patients receive one-on-one, dedicated, customized care for the aesthetic surgery patient. We have the ability to transfer patients to the hospital. Having performed surgeries in our own surgery center since 1999, I haven't had to use this option, but it is there. I do have patients for whom I recommend a hospital setting due to certain medical conditions.

Another advantage of the accredited ambulatory surgery center is lower surgical fees for the patient. There are no extra layers of bureaucracy, so we're able to pass those savings on to the patient.

Initial Consultation with Your Surgeon

Should you opt to go forward, your next step is to select a highly regarded, experienced surgeon. This is, without a doubt, the most important part of the process. To start, consider doing a web search, or ask a trusted doctor or blepharoplasty patient for a referral.

Board certification, in my opinion, is a minimum standard. It does not, however, constitute training in a specialized area.

It is strongly recommended that you choose a surgeon who has dedicated his or her primary practice to include this particular procedure.

Ask the prospective surgeon if blepharoplasty is a major focus of his or her practice. If the surgeon or the staff can look you in the eye and say *yes* without batting an eye, you are most likely dealing with a highly skilled and experienced doctor.

Such doctors are likely educating others on a national or even international level and are considered leaders in the field. This is the level of competency and care you want for your surgery.

Once you schedule an appointment, consider what information you would like to know about the surgery and the doctor performing it.

Don't be reluctant to ask for the surgeon's credentials or blepharoplasty experience. Feel free to bring photos or other visuals to help you communicate your concerns.

A confident and competent surgeon will appreciate this opportunity to assure you and put you at ease. It's also a wonderful way to build rapport, facilitate greater communication, and increase the likelihood that your expectations will be understood and met.

Depending on where you live, there may not be a thriving local practice or many to choose from, but don't let that get in your way. Consider the option of traveling to the best surgical practice for an initial consultation, which, in most instances, will be worth the additional time and relatively modest consultation fee of about $150.

Once you arrive at the office, you will be given paper work to fill out prior to your preconsult with the doctor's staff. You may also have the option, as in my practice, to download and print out necessary patient information forms from the practice's website, complete them ahead of time, and bring them to your appointment.

In my practice these include the following:

New-Patient Information Form
New-Patient Medical-History Form
HIPAA Contract*
HIPAA Notice of Privacy Practice*
Preop Anesthesia Form
Patient Medicine-Reconciliation Form
Postop Instructions for Plastic Surgery

---

*These forms explain your rights under HIPAA—the United States Health Insurance Portability and Accountability Act of 1996—regarding how your medical information may be used and disclosed and how you can get access to this information.

Take a Look Around

While you wait to meet with the surgeon, take a look around the office. Does it exude competence and caring? Do you feel at ease? Is the waiting room clean and comfortable? Is the staff courteous and professional? Are there articles about the doctor, videos from local and national media, certificates of board approval, professional journal articles, or perhaps thank-you cards from previous patients that assure you are in a first-class practice?

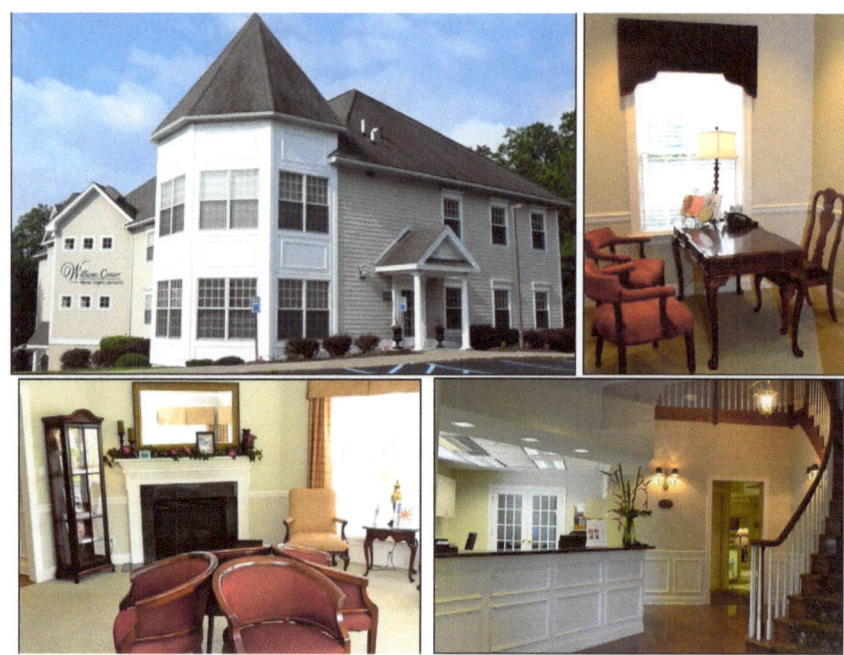

It's not just about décor, environmental aesthetics or first impressions; such efforts demonstrate the physician's commitment to provide you and all his or her patients with the best possible experience.

Blepharoplasty-Consultation Checklist

I have included a helpful blepharoplasty-consultation checklist to take with you to your consultation. Although a good surgeon will cover all the necessary points, it is best to have a written list so nothing important is missed—especially as you may be understandably nervous during the consultation.

As you consider the best surgeon for your blepharoplasty, there are important questions you want the surgeon or his or her staff to answer. The consultation checklist below includes such questions and provides an easy way to remember them as well as keep track of a surgeon's responses.

Plastic-surgeon's name:

Office phone number:

Date of consultation:

Time of appointment:

Credentials

Are you board certified?	Yes or No
American Board of Facial Plastic and Reconstructive Surgery?	Yes or No
American Board of Plastic Surgery?	Yes or No
Additional board certifications: _____	

Blepharoplasty Experience

How long have you been performing blepharoplasty procedures?	
How many blepharoplasty procedures have you performed?	
How many times do you perform blepharoplasty procedures in an average year?	
Do you teach other surgeons blepharoplasty surgery?	Yes or No
Have you been published on the subject of blepharoplasty?	Yes or No

Surgical Procedures

Ask to see before and after photos of some of the doctor's blepharoplasty patients.

Can I speak with one of your past blepharoplasty patients?   Yes   or   No

Where will the surgery be performed? _____

Is the surgical facility an accredited ambulatory surgery center? Yes   or   No

If yes, by which accrediting agencies? _____

Feel free to ask for a tour of the surgery facilities.

At which hospitals do you have admitting privileges?

_____

Medical Conditions and Medications

Write down any of your existing medical conditions to discuss with the plastic surgeon. Also make a list of the medications you are taking, and don't forget to include vitamins and other supplements as they can cause interactions with anesthesia or other medications. I have included a list of medications, vitamins, and supplements to avoid on page 40 to help with this process.

Blepharoplasty Costs

What is the cost for the surgery?

Does this include the costs of anesthesia, and surgical facilities.? Yes   or   No

If not, what are the additional costs?

Do I need to buy any medications before or after the surgery?   Yes   or   No

Do I need to buy medical supplies (ice packs, eye drops, etc.)?

If so, what will they cost?

What kind of pain medications will I be given?

What are they, and what might they cost?

Who can I talk to about my payment options, including insurance coverage and financing?

Anesthesia

What type of anesthesia will you use? _____

Who will administer the anesthesia? _____

What are his or her credentials? _____

The Blepharoplasty Procedure

Describe the procedure, and provide any imaging or diagrams that will help me understand it.

_____

How do you remember what was discussed during my consultation?

_____

What complications can occur?

_____

Postoperative Care

Are there any special instructions I should follow once I get home?   Yes   or   No

Are they available online?   Yes   or   No

What should I be on the alert for after surgery that might indicate a need to call you?

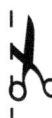

You will be given a consent form for the CGI. Be sure to read this carefully so you fully understand all the points listed on it.

During the consultation, with the aid of imaging, diagrams, and hand sketches, the surgeon will give you a comprehensive overview of the blepharoplasty procedure and discuss your options, such as where you would prefer the incisions to be placed. Most experienced surgeons have a portfolio of before and after pictures of their blepharoplasty operations that demonstrate their skill and expertise. These pictures can help you and your surgeon "get on the same page" about what's an achievement in cases similar to yours. A good practice can also arrange for you to speak with patients to discuss their experience with the practice and the surgery as you decide whether or not to go forward.

I've noticed that some patients worry that I may forget the particulars of their case, given the span of time between their consultation and the date of surgery may be several weeks apart. For this reason I let them know during our preoperative appointment that I take very detailed notes, thoroughly review imaging photos, and then design a specific plan for their surgery.

Fees, Costs, and Payment Options

At the end of the consultation, you will meet with the surgeon's staff to review fees, costs, and payment options.

Blepharoplasty costs can vary widely. According to the American Society of Plastic Surgeons, the average cost of lower lid blepharoplasty with fat transfer is $5600 which includes operating room and anesthesia fees. A brow lift runs about $8600, which also includes operating room and anesthesia fees.

The total costs depend on whether you are correcting both sets of lids (upper *and* lower) or one set of lids (upper *or* lower). For example, our sliver procedure (upper lid only) runs about $2,300 when done in the office and an additional $1,300 if done in our surgical facility. The cost of an upper and lower blepharoplasty and fat transfers is approximately $7300 which includes operating room and anesthesia fees.

When choosing a board-certified plastic surgeon for eyelid surgery, remember that the surgeon's experience and your comfort with him or her are just as important as the cost of the surgery.

If you are certain blepharoplasty is for you and you have chosen the right surgeon, you can schedule your surgery along with preop requirements, such as an EKG or physical examination. Remember, you are not obligated to commit to the surgery at the end of the initial consulting. If you need more time to think over your decision, by all means take it. You owe it to yourself to consider any reservations.

You will not be the first or last person to opt for a nonsurgical approach after a consultation. The key to a successful consultation is thorough preparation. Good communication between you and your surgeon will increase the likelihood of getting the look you want. Speak up and take an active role in the consult and in the process that follows.

Chapter 4

Before Your Blepharoplasty (Preoperative Preparation)

During your initial consultation, your surgeon should discuss with you any potential complications that may occur with eyelid surgery, such as bleeding, difficulty in completely closing the eyes, dry eyes, infection, pulling down of the lower lids, slight asymmetry in healing or scarring, swelling at the corners of the eyelids, temporary blurred or double vision, and whiteheads near your incision lines.

At your preoperative appointment, your doctor's staff should give you instructions to follow before and after your blepharoplasty surgery. These should include when to schedule your next appointment, swelling and pain medications, and recommended supplements for faster healing.

Some surgeons recommend taking bromelain (a protein extract), vitamin C (ascorbic acid), as well as *Arnica* (a natural herb) two weeks before and after surgery as they can decrease swelling and bruising. It's best to obtain all prescriptions and medications before your surgery so they are ready when you return home.

Again, be sure to inform your doctor about your daily medications (bring a list for easy recall) so he or she can advise you on which of these must be avoided and which can be taken (with just a sip of water) the morning of your surgery.

If you are taking prescription blood thinners, such as Coumadin and Plavix, do not stop taking them without a discussion with the prescribing physician. Be sure to also discuss any vitamins, herbal supplements, or diet pills as they may contain elements that thin the blood and interfere with anesthesia.

It is very important that the contents of any over-the-counter preparations be checked carefully as well. Many headache preparations, cold remedies, and "hangover cures" contain aspirin (chemical name for aspirin is acetylsalicylic acid) or ibuprofen and should be avoided two weeks before the surgery. You can substitute Tylenol occasionally for the products above.

Examples of Drugs Containing Aspirin (acetylsalicylic acid)

Examples of drugs containing salicylates are as follows:

Acetidine	Coricidin	Excedrin	Menadob	Robassisal
Alka-Seltzer	Cephalgesic	Feldene	Mobidin	Roxiprin
Amigesic	Cheracol Caps	Fenoprin	Monogesic	Rufin
Anacin	Clinoril	Fiorinol	Nabumetone	Saleto
Anahist	Congesprin	Froben	Nalfon	Salflex
Anaprox	Children's ASA	Flurbiprofen	Norgesic	Sine Off
Anaproxin	Choline Salicylate	Gelprin	Norwich EX	Sine Aid
Ansaid	Cope	Genpril	Ocufen	Soma Compound
APC	Corticosteroids	Genprin	Orudis	Suldinac
Argesic`	Coumadin	Goody's Body	Oruvail	Synalgos DC
Arthra G	Daypro	Haltran	Oxyphenbutazone	
Arthropan	Depakote	Halfprin	Oxybuta	Tanacetum
Ascodeen	Dilofenac	Ibuprin	Oxyprozin	Trandate
Ascriptin	Dipyridamole	Ketoprofen	Pamprin	Trigesic
Aspergum	Disalcid	Ketorolac	Peptol Bismol	Trental
Aspirin	Divalproex	Lortab ASA	Pecodan	Trilisate
Baby Aspirin	Doan's Pill	Liquiprin	Persantin	Tusal
Bayer	Dolobid	Magan	Phenaphen	Vanquish
BC Powder	Dristan	MG Sallicylate	Piroxicam	Voltaren
Bromo-Quinine	Easprin	Meclofenamate	Ponstel	Warfarin
Bromo-Selzter	Ecotrin	Meclofen	Prednisone	WillowBark
Brufen	Emprazil	Medipren	Quagesic	Zactrin
Bufferin	Empirin	Mefenamic	Relafen	
Butazolidin	Endodan	Midol	Rexolate	

Examples of aspirin-related products (Ibuprofen, Indomethacin, Naproxen, Tolmetin)

Advil	Naprosyn	Indocin	Tolectin
Aleve	Nuprin	Motrin	Toradol

You can substitute *TYLENOL* **occasionally** for the products above, however, avoid taking them *daily* for 2 weeks prior to surgery.

As I said before, if you are taking regular prescription medications for high blood pressure, diabetes, heart disease, or asthma, *please* check with your doctor before disrupting your routinely scheduled medications.

Supplements—It is important to discontinue the use of the following supplements two weeks prior to surgery, and for up to two weeks after surgery:

- Bilberry ▪ Cayenne ▪ CoQ10 ▪ Dong quai ▪ Echinacea ▪ Feverfew ▪ Fish oil Caps ▪ Garlic ▪ Ginger ▪ Ginseng ▪ Ginkgo biloba ▪ Hawthorne ▪ Kava kava ▪ Licorice root ▪ Ma huang (ephedra) ▪ Melatonin ▪ Red clover ▪ Valerian ▪ St. John's Wort ▪ Vitamin E ▪ Yohimbe ▪ Multivitamins

Alcohol—Ideally, abstain from drinking a week or two prior to and after surgery as this can promote healing.

Nicotine—Nicotine interferes with healing by reducing blood flow. Avoid smoking, as well as gums and patches that contain nicotine, for at least two weeks prior to your procedure.

Increase fluids a few days prior to surgery. We find that patients recover faster from anesthesia when they are well hydrated, and we encourage them to increase their water intake a few days before surgery. Just remember—do not eat or drink any food or liquids after midnight the day before the surgery, including water, candy, mints, or gum. You can brush your teeth.

The night before surgery, feel free to wash your hair and face. Don't apply makeup on the morning of the surgery. Leave all jewelry at home, including rings, earrings, watches, and any piercings. Contact lenses should not be worn the day of the surgery. Eyeglasses are acceptable and can be brought into the operating room with you.

You'll want to wear comfortable clothing, such as yoga pants or sweatpants and a shirt or sweater with front closures to avoid pulling it over your head.

Risks and Complications of Anesthesia

Anesthesia is very safe, especially when administered by an anesthesiologist or nurse anesthetist, but safe does not mean there is no risk. You need to understand what the risks are and tell your surgeon if you have any heart or respiratory problems. Other underlying problems, such as liver or kidney disease, can interfere with anesthesia and raise the chance of an adverse event. Smokers are more likely to have problems with anesthesia than people who do not smoke.

Remember, thousands of people have anesthesia every day. Most of the associated risks are very small and unlikely to happen. The vast majority of people undergoing surgery with any type of anesthesia do just fine.

This information is not meant to alarm you but rather to inform you so you can make a well-educated decision about your anesthesia.

Fasting before Surgery

Your stomach needs to be empty in the event you become nauseated during or immediately after your surgery. This also means no breath mints, lozenges, or gum. If you must take a medication the morning of your surgery, consult with your surgeon first. It is important to follow your surgeon's preoperative instructions to avoid any problems.

The Day of Your Surgery

On the day of your surgery, your surgeon will review the details captured in your chart from previous consultations and talk with you about your agreed-on goals for the procedure. At our center we do this after the patient has checked in. I also let my patients know their photos and images will be displayed on the monitors in the operating room as we use them as a guide since patients tend to look a little different lying down than in an upright position. I feel it is an important consideration for achieving the optimal and best outcome for a cosmetic procedure. These help me refer to the subtler aspects of their eyes, which may be less obvious during the procedure due to swelling from local anesthesia and from the patient lying flat on the table.

Next, a nurse or other health professional will start an IV with fluids that may contain antibiotics. Blepharoplasty is usually done in an outpatient ambulatory surgical center unless you opt for the sliver technique (see page 21), which is performed in the doctor's office. Depending on the amount and location of tissue being removed, blepharoplasty takes about an hour or less. During this time you will be pain-free, relaxed, and kept still thanks to anesthesia, which is administered by a certified registered nurse anesthetist (CRNA) or an anesthesiologist (a medical doctor who specializes in anesthesia). Your surgeon will inject numbing medication into your eyelid skin while you are sedated.

During the procedure your surgeon will make precise markings based on a customized and specific preoperative evaluation of your underlying facial-muscle and bone structure and the symmetry of your eyebrows. Sutures are carefully applied to smooth and reconfigure areas around eyelids. After upper-lid surgery, no dressing is used above the lids so vision is not impeded.

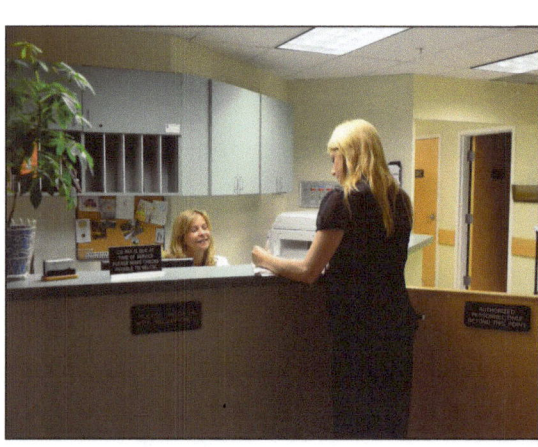
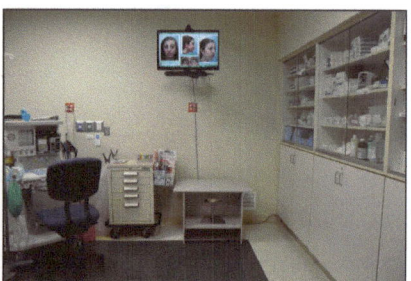
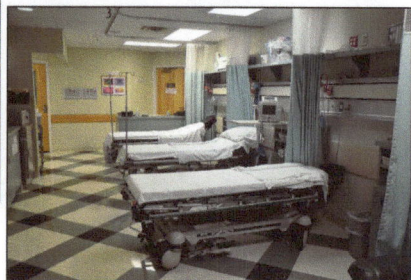

If a brow-lift procedure is also done at the same time, incisions are made in the scalp area to tighten the skin and lift the underlying brow tissue. A carbon dioxide (CO_2) laser or deep chemical peel may also be done at this time to enhance the procedure by resurfacing skin and smoothing out any remaining wrinkles in the eyelid and eyebrow area.

As the local anesthetic wears off and the nerves wake up from being "asleep," the area will feel sore for a few hours. Typically, acetaminophen (Tylenol) should be taken on a proactive basis (every four to six hours) and is usually adequate for this temporary discomfort. However, some patients require prescription pain medication.

By the evening of the surgery, pain is minimal. Most patients do not need any pain medicine by the next morning. By the second day, discomfort is minimal or no longer experienced.

Chapter 5

After Your Blepharoplasty Surgery (Postoperative Procedures)

After eyelid surgery some tightness and soreness of the eyelids can occur. Patients should keep their heads elevated as much as possible during the first few days and regularly apply cold compresses to help reduce swelling and bruising. Most patients do not complain of discomfort but often describe it as being sore and feeling like a small paper cut. This can be alleviated with a small amount of antibiotic over the incision. Dryness, itchiness, burning, excessive tearing, and sensitivity to light can occur during the first week. If you experience blurriness, use less antibiotic ointment as this is very likely the cause. Also you can use a few drops of over-the-counter saline eye solution by tilting your head back *without* pulling on the eyelids. It typically takes ten days for the bruising to fade.

Patients can usually resume reading within a day or two. Work and most normal activities, including alcohol consumption, may be resumed within seven to ten days, while contact lenses may be worn after two weeks. More strenuous activities should be avoided for about three weeks.

If you are concerned about anything you consider significant, do not hesitate to call your doctor.

General Postop Instructions following Blepharoplasty

1. Sleep on your back or side with head elevated above your chest.

2. Blepharoplasty usually involves little or no postoperative pain. If you experience significant sharp or dull pain that persists, notify your doctor's office immediately.

3. Cold compresses over your eyes should be used every twenty to thirty minutes for up to seventy-two hours to minimize swelling.

4. It is quite common to have asymmetrical swelling. This does not affect the outcome of surgery.

5. Do not wear contact lenses for at least two weeks. Pulling on the eyelids while inserting or removing lenses may interfere with precise incision healing. Glasses may be worn at any time.

6. Do not use mascara, eyeliner, or eye shadow until approved by your doctor (usually ten to fourteen days). Minimal makeup applied to any bruising of the lower lid is acceptable at any time, but do not pull on the lids or incisions.

7. Any apparent redness of the whites of the eyeball is a mild form of bruising and will subside during the early healing process. Occasionally, during the first week after surgery, a small amount of blood may be discharged from the eyes. This is not unusual as it is a result of the blood collecting during surgery and releasing. It is likely to happen once and pass quickly.

8. Do not engage in vigorous exercise or sports for at least three weeks or until approved by your doctor.

9. A follow-up appointment with your doctor is usually made for six days after surgery.

10. It is normal to feel slight itching and tightness of the eyelids during the early healing period. Avoid salty foods before and after surgery as they can cause increased swelling and pain.

11. If you are prescribed an antibiotic after your surgery, remember to take it with food.

Postop Instructions following Transconjunctival Blepharoplasty

(Eyelid Surgery with External Incisions)

1. Follow the postop instructions for blepharoplasty.
2. Clean the incision line with diluted hydrogen peroxide, and then apply an antibacterial ointment (Bacitracin). Use both products sparingly; avoid getting them in your eyes.
3. Stitches are usually removed six days after surgery, depending on the extent of surgery.
4. *Optional*: Two weeks postop, you may begin taking ibuprofen, such as Advil, or Aleve (as directed). Take until all redness or inflammation is gone—but not longer than three weeks.

Chapter 6

Additional Postoperative Recommendations

Rest quietly in bed (or in a reclining chair) with your head elevated (above the level of your heart) for the first forty-eight to seventy-two hours after surgery. Continue sleeping elevated for approximately one week, and, if possible, on your back for a few weeks afterward. It is common to have low energy levels following surgery. Unnecessary activity will encourage swelling, discomfort, and bleeding. Minimize all activities for several days until these symptoms resolve.

Resist using your recovery period to catch up on errands, exercise, or home projects. You need rest.

When and What to Eat

In most cases a healthy appetite will return within twenty-four to forty-eight hours of anesthesia. Start eating when you feel hungry. Consider light liquids (broth, ginger ale, crackers, toast, etc.), and progress slowly to regular foods. Increase fluids such as water and fruit juices (no citrus fruits). Avoid alcohol, nicotine, and caffeine as these will dramatically slow the healing process.

First Postoperative Appointment

Your first return appointment will be approximately six to seven days following surgery. At this time, your physician will remove the stitches from the eyelid-surgery procedure. We usually take a set of photos at this appointment for comparative purposes.

Some patients experience discouragement or mild depression after cosmetic surgery. It is natural to be concerned when your face is a bit swollen and bruised.

After you are home for a few days, you should be comfortable watching television or reading. However, you won't be able to wear contact lenses for a few weeks after your blepharoplasty.

It's advisable to keep your activity level to a minimum for three to five days after surgery. To keep your blood pressure down, you should avoid strenuous activities for three weeks to one month. This includes heavy lifting, bending, and participating in sports activities. Also to be avoided are things that cause fluid retention, such as high-fat, salty foods and excessive amounts of alcohol. Don't avoid drinking water though! Proper fluid intake is important to your health and healing.

Most patients feel comfortable going out in public after a week or two. When you resume social activities and return to work really depends on you. The average patient returns to work or social activities in seven to fourteen days.

At about two weeks, you can start with aerobic activities; however, avoid anything involving contact for three weeks. After this period most patients are healed and can get back to contact activities, knowing that any direct hit to the eyes could result in additional surgery.

Caring for the Eyes

After upper- and lower-blepharoplasty surgery, the eyelids typically feel tight; accompanying soreness may be treated with analgesics. For the first couple of days following the surgery, the incisions should be treated with ointment to keep them lubricated. Cold compresses can be placed on the eyes to reduce swelling as well. Saline eye drops can be used occasionally during the first week if they feel dry. However, if the dryness persists, speak to your doctor. (Do not use redness-removing eye drops.)

During this time, patients should avoid any activities that may dry up the eyes, including excessive reading, watching television, wearing contacts, and using a computer. Swelling and bruising can be minimized by keeping the head elevated as much as possible during the first few days of recovery. Patients may feel well enough to resume normal activities around the tenth day of recovery.

Approximately 90 percent of upper-eyelid blepharoplasty patients see little or no bruising four to five days after surgery. Most patients have only a little wisp of a bruise under each eye. Lower-lid blepharoplasty can cause slightly more bruising, especially if you have fat transfers, and take a little more time to disappear.

Camouflaging cosmetic products can be used to help cover any remaining bruising and are often available from your plastic surgeon's office as well as many places where makeup is sold. Just make sure you check with your surgeon to ensure that your products won't cause an adverse reaction.

Healing after Blepharoplasty

Healing after surgery takes time. Your incision lines will eventually fade and become nearly invisible. Until that happens, you can expect that the incision line to be pinkish. The pinkness can persist for six months or so. The sun can make incision lines appear more prominent, so protecting them from the sun is essential. For the first couple of weeks following the surgery, dark sunglasses are recommended to protect the eyes from irritation caused by the sun and wind. Patients may notice that their eyes tire easily for the first few weeks of the recovery period.

How Long Does Blepharoplasty Last?

Blepharoplasty has some of the longest-lasting results—so much so that after you have one, you probably won't need to get another ever again. This is not to say that once you recover from your blepharoplasty, your eyelids will stay exactly as they are for the rest of your life. Plastic surgery can improve your appearance, but it can't prevent you from aging, and your face will continue to change as the years go by.

The changes made during your eyelid surgery should be more or less permanent. Any fat removed from the eyelids, for example, will not grow back (even if you gain weight). Bags under the eyes and hoods over the eyes shouldn't appear again, either. There is a chance that the brow will descend later on, which can cause new folds to appear on the upper eyelids—but this is generally something that should be dealt with through a brow lift or facelift, not blepharoplasty.

Many experts will say blepharoplasty lasts from ten to fifteen years, but in my experience, this is not a hard-and-fast rule. While some retouching may be necessary, most people who undergo blepharoplasty once will never have to do it again—especially if you go to a qualified surgeon who gets it right the first time.

Chapter 7

Nonsurgical Eyelid Procedures

A surgical eye-lift can definitely take years off your face, but it is not for everyone. While the "no-knife" options cannot produce the full effect of surgery, cosmetic alternatives to surgical procedures can give your eyes a noticeable boost.

Procedures like Botox injections and laser resurfacing are quite effective. Other prescription medicine injections like Juvéderm, Restylane, Radiesse, Perlane, and Sculptra can improve the appearance by correcting crow's-feet, smile lines, bunny lines (wrinkles on the side of the upper nose), forehead lines, and furrows between the eyebrows.

Even daily use of a good moisturizer made especially for the eyes can contribute to a younger, more refreshed appearance.

Botox and Dysport

Botox is a drug made from a neurotoxin produced by the bacterium *Clostridium botulinum* called botulinum toxin. It is used medically to treat certain muscular conditions and remove wrinkles by temporarily relaxing muscles. Botox takes up to seven to ten days to work, while Dysport, an injectable wrinkle relaxer similar to Botox, works more quickly.

In our plastic-surgery practice, we inject the smallest and most effective amount of medication possible in order to relax the muscles of the face without hindering normal facial expressions.

Some practices charge a set fee each time a patient returns for an injection visit. However, at our center we often use less medication than in previous visits as the muscles are already relaxed or weakened. This means we do not inject the same amount of medication each time if it is not needed, which reduces the cost for our patients. Botox injections may seem like a fairly simple procedure, but the delivery of consistent results requires an experienced practitioner.

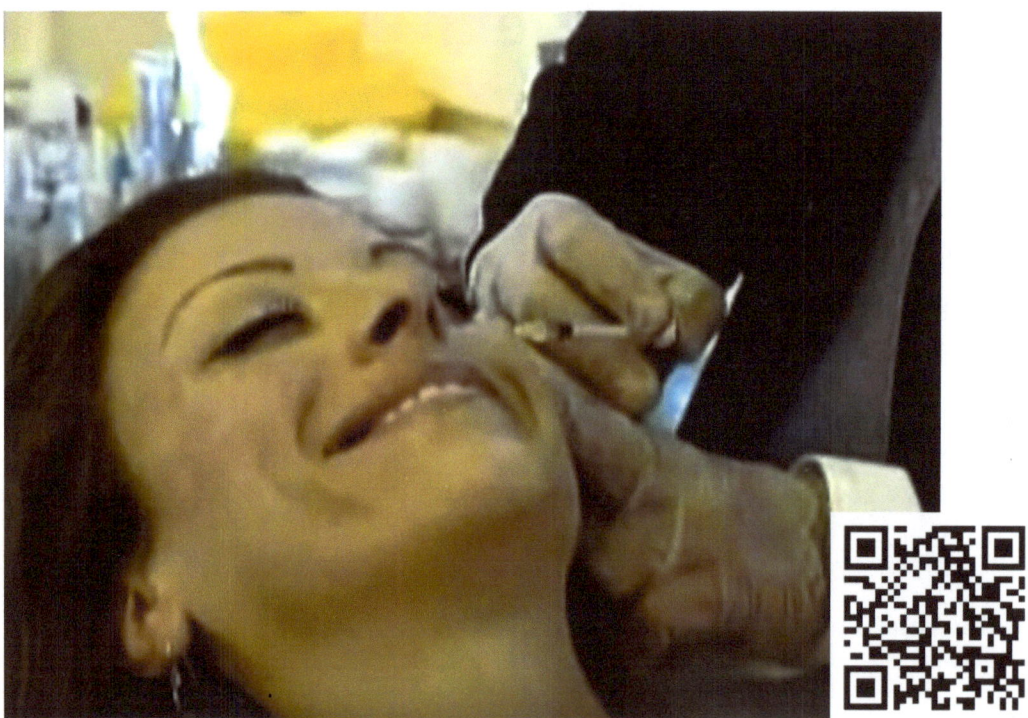

Volume and Fillers

Products like Voluma, Juvéderm, and Restylane offer their own volumizing options for the midface and the glabella—the area of skin between the eyebrows.

Tear-trough fillers, such as Restylane, help to reduce the bags, circles, dark shadows, and puffiness associated with wear and tear around the eyes. At our center, for the right candidate, a Restylane tear-trough procedure is quick and simple—with minimal swelling and bruising of the injection site.

Here are the complaints we hear most often and how we treat them nonsurgically.

- Wrinkles and furrows:
  Tiny crow's-feet to deep lines can be virtually erased by muscle-relaxing injections, like Botox and Dysport, and resurfacing lasers and chemical-peel procedures. Also, fillers can help here. And again, a good eye moisturizer can soften the appearance of wrinkles around the eyes.
- Drooping or hooded eyelids:
  Injecting Botox to relax your brow muscles can lift heavy eyelids and help open up your eyes so they look more youthful and awake.
- Hollow under-eye areas resulting from fat loss or dark under-eye circles:
  Filler injections can plump up the recesses around the eyes as well as plump up cheeks, shortening the distance from the lower lid to the top of the cheek, which reflects the facial structure of a younger person.
- Puffy under eyes caused by fat:
  Fillers can be injected around the puffy areas to camouflage them. However, a surgical approach is far more effective in addressing the issue.

Nonsurgical Brow Treatments

As discussed earlier, one of the hardest hit spots during the aging process is the forehead and brow, and it's one of the hardest areas to treat with Botox or Dysport. Brow-lift surgery is probably the best treatment option to soften deep lines and hooding skin in this area.

That being said, injections placed strategically in the muscles of the brow can lift them to a more natural-looking position and alleviate pressure and sagging. While this could inadvertently drop the brow, causing a droopy-eye appearance, it can easily be corrected with an injection or with Alphagan eye drops, which stimulate a second set of muscles and lift the eyelid muscle. Some patients are happy to repeat Botox treatments at regular intervals to maintain these results, while others use it as a preview of what surgery could offer them.

Getting Ready for Botox and Other Injectables

While many patients have little to do before Botox or Dysport injections, there are some ways to minimize posttreatment complications and to achieve the best possible results.

One of the most important things you can do before having Dysport or Botox injections is research the cosmetic injector you're considering for the procedure. Botox, in the wrong hands, can produce poor results that aren't quite what you expected. Legally, any doctor, nurse practitioner, or registered nurse, under the direction of a physician, can perform the injections, but that doesn't necessarily mean he or she has adequate training or experience with such products.

Ideally, you want a doctor or cosmetic injector who is under the direction of someone who specializes in plastic surgery and cosmetic treatments. Don't hesitate to ask how long the doctor or cosmetic injector has been doing injections, how many they perform in a week, and what special training they have received. You can also ask to speak with others in the practice who have had injections or review before and after photos of their work.

Things to Tell Your Doctor or Cosmetic Injector

The consultation before a Botox injection is similar to other medical consultations. Your cosmetic injector will likely recommend that you avoid taking medicines that thin the blood, such as aspirin, for a few days before the injection. Taking blood thinners increases your risk for bruising and bleeding afterward. However, always check with your primary physician before stopping any medication. See the chart on pages 39 and 40 for other medications and supplements, including some vitamins, that thin the blood.

At our center we discovered the pulsed dye laser can minimize or eliminate bruising almost overnight, and we offer this to patients, if needed, at no charge.

You'll also want to let the injector know about any allergies, such as latex, or any history of adverse reactions to injectables.

Eating, Drinking, and Other Habits

Your cosmetic injector may also recommend avoiding alcohol a few days prior to injections. Generally, it's a good idea to do any daily exercise or workout before your Botox injections as you want to wait at least a day before exercising again.

Timing Your Injections

When it comes to Botox or Dysport, timing matters. If you are having the injections in advance of a special occasion, schedule the treatment well in advance. The injections typically last at least three months. You want to give them time to take effect and time for any side effects, such as redness and bruising, to diminish. Two or three weeks before a big event is time enough for Botox injections to take effect (sooner for Dysport) and for any side effects to fade.

About Injectables

Muscle Relaxer (Botox, Dysport)
- Purified substance from bacteria that helps relax muscles so sagging lids, brow furrows, and crepe-like skin look more taut
- $200 to $600 for the eye area
- Lasts for three to four months
- Mild soreness, slight bruising

Hyaluronic-Acid-Gel Filler (like Restylane, Juvéderm, and Voluma)
- The synthetic version of a naturally occurring protein-sugar compound found in skin. It binds to water and plumps facial folds or fills in under-eye hollows.
- $500 to $1,000 per injection
- Lasts for nine months to two years and sometimes longer
- Minimal discomfort with a topical anesthetic or nerve block
- Possible swelling and bruising (disguisable with makeup)

Skin Care for the Eyes

While some facial plastic surgeons focus strictly on aesthetics through surgery, we take a multifaceted approach to each treatment plan at our practice. Skin care, specifically medicated skin-care products, can optimize and help everyone's skin look and feel more youthful, whether they choose nonsurgical or surgical procedures.

The array of medically crafted formulas, however, can prove overwhelming for some patients. The market is flooded with creams that promise to erase or reduce wrinkles or improve the color, texture, and tone of your skin. The question is, what really works?

The following information is aimed at providing patients with an overview of the various skin-care products available and their effectiveness. While some are available without a prescription, others require a prescription, such as those I've formulated into a creamier, nonirritating base, and contain active ingredients scientifically proven to reverse sun damage and stimulate collagen production. These prescription-strength creams are most effective and should be the foundation of your skin-care regime.

I recommend a consultation with a highly trained, skin-care medical professional who can develop a daily routine specific to your skin-care needs.

Medicated Skin-Care Products

Medicated skin-care products containing tretinoin, the active ingredient in Retin-A, are the key to treating and preventing lines, wrinkles, and skin creases. Since such products do require a prescription, you should use these products carefully. Be sure to read package directions and heed any warnings regarding possible allergies, side effects, and other consequences. Human nature often thinks more is better; however, with Retin-A products a little goes a long way.

Alpha-hydroxy cream uses carboxylic and hydroxyl acid (the same chemicals used in dermatological chemical peels) to exfoliate the skin so that it can fully benefit from serums and moisturizers. Think of your skin as a raisin or dry sponge. When you add water, it plumps up and softens the lines or rough spots. If your skin is not properly exfoliated, your moisturizer will have little effect. Again, you want to use these diligently while avoiding overuse as it may cause irritation.

Eye-cream products can help alleviate the effects of sleep deprivation or sun damage underneath the eyes. Eye-care products should be applied carefully to avoid any direct contact with the eye itself.

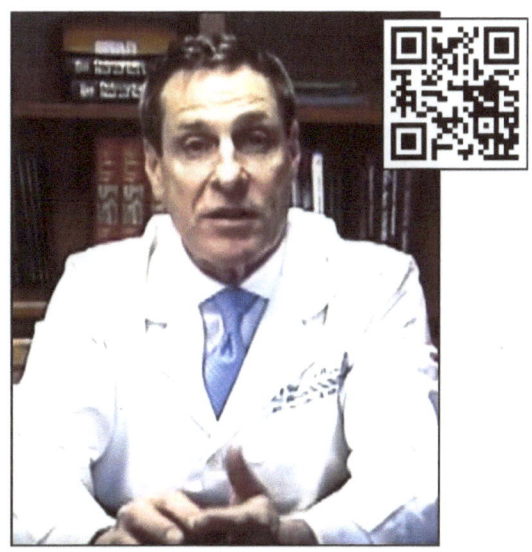

Step-by-Step Recommended Skin-Care Regime

1. Cleanse

    When used twice daily, a skin cleanser can effectively maintain a moisture balance in the skin conducive to a fresh, healthy appearance. Face washes are formulated for many types of skin, including oily or acne-prone, normal, and dry. Specialized product lines may cater to a wider range of skin conditions and issues. A cleanser helps to remove impurities from the skin, including daily pollutants and cosmetics. Men are encouraged to use many of the same skin-care products as women, including facial cleansers.

2. **Exfoliate**

Cell renewal is paramount to skin health and aesthetics. To speed up this process and ensure new cells are always present, exfoliants remove older skin cells, soften the skin, and create a more uniform complexion. Exfoliation also clears debris from the pores, lessening the appearance of blackheads. The gritty particles in these skin treatments may be natural or synthetic and vary in size. Because of the abrasive nature of the product, many skin scrubs are not suggested for everyday use.

3. **Tone, Tone, Tone**

Once the skin has been cleansed and exfoliated, the next step in the skin-care regimen is the application of toner. Typically offered in liquid formulation, this product is not rinsed from the skin. A toner may be formulated to combat acne, moisturize the skin, or treat the skin in other ways. This product also removes the last bit of makeup that may be remaining on the skin. The ideal application involves a cotton pad or cotton ball and enough toner to smooth over the entire face. The skin should feel moisturized but not dripping wet.

4. **Serums**

Serums and moisturizers are not interchangeable products as the former is a power-packed, concentrated treatment and the latter has the main duty of hydrating the skin. Typically, serums are slightly thicker than moisturizers and have a gel consistency. A facial serum may be designed to combat lines and wrinkles or other signs of aging.

These treatments offer the strongest, most effective ingredients that are comparable to prescription-strength skin care and are quickly absorbed by the skin. Customizing them for your skin is recommended as there are many formulas available.

5. **Eye Creams**

The eyes may exhibit signs of aging in people as early as their twenties, which is why some eye creams have been developed to prevent this. Some patients still question the use of a separate treatment for the eye area and often skip this step in their skin-care regiment until they learn of its importance. The eye area surrounding these vital organs of vision is very sensitive with some of the thinnest skin on your body. Nonspecific products may contain ingredients that irritate the eyes or are untested for use around the eyes. Since the skin is thin and the eyes are involved in many facial movements and expressions, products designed for the overall face may be insufficient in treating the signs of aging in this area. Remember, too, not every eye cream is developed for the creases commonly known as crow's-feet. Some treat dark, under-eye circles and under-eye bags. It is best to consult a medical professional for eye treatments who addresses your specific concerns.

6. **Moisturize**

Once a serum and eye cream have been fully absorbed by the skin, a moisturizer can be smoothed over the face. Moisturizers not only soften the skin but may also contain treatment ingredients. Facial hydrators are created in a wide variety of formulations to suit the needs of the various types of skin. This promotes optimal skin health and long-lasting comfort throughout the day and night. While other steps in the skin-care process may only be performed once daily, it is typically advised that patients moisturize their skin two times each day, once in the morning and once at night. For daytime, a lighter facial lotion with an SPF is ideal, while at night a nurturing treatment cream can be applied.

Eyelashes and Aging

Unfortunately, thinning eyelashes are part of the aging process. Eyelash growth has four stages: growth, resting, shedding, and regrowth. Your lashes continuously cycle through these four stages. And as we age, eyelash follicles (the openings in the skin through which the lash grows) can slow or stop producing new lashes altogether.

Other Reasons for Thinning Eyelashes

Another reason for thinning lashes is simple irritation. If you rub your eyes constantly, you eventually irritate the follicles. Other factors, including genetics, medications, and certain medical conditions, can also cause thinning lashes.

Latisse Eyelash Treatment

Allergan, the makers of Botox Cosmetic, makes the only FDA-approved solution to inadequate eyelashes, called Latisse, that causes lashes to grow in thicker, darker, and longer.

Latisse seems to prolong the active growth phase of your lashes. The majority of patients will begin to see a subtle difference in lashes at eight weeks, a noticeable difference at twelve weeks, and often a dramatic difference at sixteen weeks. If you stop using Latisse, your lashes will gradually return to their previous appearance over the course of several weeks to several months.

Available only through a prescription, a nurse practitioner or physician will discuss with you the benefits and side effects of Latisse. Not everyone is a candidate for Latisse, so it's important to tell your provider if you have risk factors for glaucoma, have been diagnosed with or are taking medication for eye pressure problems, or may be allergic to one of Latisse's ingredients.

It is also important to contact your physician if you have developed any new eye conditions or reactions while using Latisse. Your physician can safely assess whether or not you should discontinue the use of Latisse. Possible side effects of Latisse include eye itching, irritation, dryness, redness, and skin darkening of the eyelids. There is also a chance of an increase in brown iris pigmentation for patients with blue, gray, or green eyes, which is likely to be permanent.

Application

Latisse is applied once every night on a clean face free of makeup and contacts removed (if applicable), using the applicators supplied with your bottle of Latisse. These special applicators are designed to properly apply the Latisse and are sterile and disposable, reducing the potential for contamination and infection. Latisse is applied to the upper lids *only*, and excess solution should be blotted away to prevent hair-growth occurrence outside the upper-eyelid area. Latisse should not be applied to the lower lid as it will transfer small amounts from the upper lid to the lower lid.

Chapter 8

Conclusion

Successful facial plastic surgery requires good communication between patient and surgeon. It requires trust, based on realistic expectations and exacting medical expertise and developed in the consulting stages before surgery is performed.

I've enjoyed sharing my expertise, knowledge, and experience with you, and whatever you ultimately decide, I hope this book has proven to be a richly informative resource. While no book can completely address all your concerns and questions, it is my hope you will take whatever remaining concerns you have to a skilled surgeon who can address your specific needs.

Chapter 9

Blepharoplasty FAQs

What is blepharoplasty?
Blepharoplasty, also known as eyelid surgery, is a surgical procedure that involves the removal of excess fat, skin, and muscle in order to correct droopiness of the upper eyelids or puffy bags of the lower eyelids. This procedure may be performed on both the upper and lower eyelids or just on one.

What causes the eyelids to sag?
Eyelid skin is the thinnest on the body and can stretch with age, creating looseness and a tired appearance. Brow and cheek sagging also contribute to the appearance of eyelid aging. Prolonged sun exposure, smoking, stress, and other environmental factors can accelerate these changes. There may be hereditary influences as well, particularly with lower-eyelid bags.

What is Asian blepharoplasty?
Asian blepharoplasty creates a crease in the eyelid. Asians have what's referred to as a "single eyelid" (with no crease), and some would prefer a "double eyelid" (one with a crease). This ethnic plastic surgery is one of the most requested procedures among Asians in the United States and abroad.

How long do the results last?

Eyelid surgery tends to be very long lasting. Many people will only undergo one eyelid-lift procedure in their lifetime as compared to a neck lift, which may need to be repeated.

Do I need to see my own doctor before a blepharoplasty?

Not necessarily. If sedation is used, basic lab tests may be required, and typically patients over the age of forty-five require a written clearance from their personal physicians.

Does eyelid surgery affect vision?

Depending on the operation, ointments or drops may be used in the eyes to help protect them, which typically results in a blurred vision for a few days. The eyes can be mildly sore, moist, or slightly dry in some cases.

Can blepharoplasty improve vision?

Sometimes a blepharoplasty can improve an individual's vision by removing the excess fat and skin that may block his or her peripheral field of vision.

Can I have an eyelid lift if I have already had laser vision correction?

Laser-vision-correction surgery is a very common procedure, and we've performed blepharoplasty on many patients who have had Lasik. We recommend waiting at least six months after having laser vision correction before undergoing blepharoplasty as such correction can lead to a temporary dryness of the surface of the eyes. An eyelid lift should only be done when the surface of the eyes is at its optimal condition.

At what age is blepharoplasty performed?

Although there is no set age when blepharoplasty is performed, most patients are thirty-five years of age and up. However, this is highly individual, and excess skin and fat around the eye area can be removed at younger than thirty-five years of age.

Will a blepharoplasty rid me of my crow's-feet wrinkles?

A blepharoplasty is not designed to remove crow's-feet but can remove the wrinkles underneath the lower eyelids. It is designed to remove the excess skin and fat from the lid areas only. There are other procedures available that are area-specific to crow's-feet complaints, such as laser treatments, which can help soften periocular (around the eye) wrinkles significantly. A qualified surgeon can determine a customized approach that meets your exact needs.

Will lower blepharoplasty help with dark circles under my eyes?

Improving the shape and configuration of the lower eyelid can improve the dark circles to some degree. If the circles are caused by shadows cast by large bags beneath the eyes or hollowness in the tear-trough area, adding volume with fat during eyelid surgery can improve the appearance of dark circles.

Restylane or Juvéderm can also fill in the tear-trough area. However, there are also many other reasons for dark circles beneath the eyes, including allergies, thin skin overlying prominent (and purple) muscle, swollen veins, hyperpigmentation (darkening) of the skin, and someone's ethnic makeup. These will not be entirely improved by lower-eyelid surgery.

How do I know if I am a good candidate for an eyelid lift?

The best candidate for blepharoplasty is a physically healthy person who is realistic in his or her expectations regarding improvement of droopiness, excess skin, or bulging fat of the upper or lower eyelids. Blepharoplasty will not correct sagging of the brows, forehead furrows, or deep lines and wrinkles. These patients may benefit from other procedures, such as a brow lift or skin resurfacing. During the initial consultation, your surgeon should recommend a customized treatment plan that specifically addresses your concerns.

How many doctors should I consult with?

Consult with as many as you need to feel completely comfortable with the doctor you choose. Some patients are able to settle on their surgeons after only one blepharoplasty consultation, while others require meeting with several surgeons before making a decision. In all cases, a surgeon specializing in facial procedures is recommended.

Are computer images used to see what I will look like after the surgery?

Like many facial plastic surgeons, I use computer-generated imagery (CGI), which is a specialized computer program that allows a surgeon to manipulate a photograph and explain and develop possible surgical goals. I find this extremely helpful in effective communication between doctor and patient. The goals of one patient may be very different from another. One of the integral parts of my practice is making sure each procedure is a fully unique event. I am not creating the same change for everyone; I am partnering with my patient to create a customized surgical plan that honors his or her unique characteristics.

What other procedures may be combined with cosmetic eyelid surgery?

A number of other cosmetic procedures may be safely performed at the same time as blepharoplasty. These include skin resurfacing, facelift, neck lift, brow or forehead lift, and others.

What are the risks or complications that can occur with blepharoplasty?

The potential complications that may occur include the following: bleeding, dry eyes, slight asymmetry in healing or scarring, swelling at the corners of the eyelids, and temporary blurred vision.

Will an eyelid lift make me look fake or overdone like some celebrities?

Eyelid surgery, when expertly performed, typically results in a natural, refreshed appearance. At our center, we take each patient's expectations into account, as well as his or her physical attributes, when performing cosmetic procedures. In the case of certain celebrities that look unnatural, they likely have had "too much" or "overly aggressive" surgery performed.

Can a brow lift correct the upper eyelids?

In some cases, elevating the brows will pull up excess upper-lid skin, so a blepharoplasty may not be needed.

Can eyelid surgery be performed at the same time as nonsurgical procedures?

Absolutely. Eyelid lifts are commonly done at the same time as Botox injections and facial fillers. In fact, many patients enjoy the benefit of sharing the downtime when having multiple procedures performed simultaneously.

Can asymmetry be a problem after cosmetic eyelid surgery?

Most people have some degree of asymmetry prior to cosmetic surgery. During surgery we work to correct asymmetries; however, the human anatomy sometimes cannot be made symmetrical because the underlying skeleton, muscles, and skin attachments are asymmetric to begin with.

Perfect geometrical symmetry may produce an unnatural or artificial look. With our patients, we use the analogy that eyes are like sisters or brothers but are not necessarily twins. Attractive, youthful asymmetry is still very acceptable, especially with a patient who had a considerable amount of asymmetry before surgery.

Does eyelid surgery hurt?

No. Local anesthesia is used, and depending on the procedure, mild sedation, either with oral or intravenous medications, can be used as a supplement. A skilled surgeon ensures that you are comfortable throughout the entire procedure.

An anesthesia provider will be responsible for administering your anesthesia or sedation. Both your surgeon and the anesthesiologist work together to determine what best suits your particular needs.

Where is the blepharoplasty procedure performed?

To ensure your safety and comfort, eyelid surgery should be performed in a state-licensed, fully accredited ambulatory surgical facility. However, the eyelid sliver procedure may be performed in your doctor's office, under local anesthesia.

What do I need to do the day before surgery?

The day before surgery, you should eat normally but avoid excessively heavy meals and foods that can lead to acid reflux. Be sure to increase your water intake as it can help you more easily recover from surgery. Most importantly, do not eat or drink anything after midnight before your procedure if you are undergoing anesthesia.

How long will the procedure take?

Depending on the specific procedure and how many eyelids are being treated, the procedure can take between forty-five and ninety minutes.

What if I smoke?

Smoking increases the risks of poor healing and infection and causes increased coughing and bleeding after cosmetic surgery and other complications. As a result we strongly recommend smokers to stop smoking for at least two weeks before surgery.

Can I continue to take my regular medications?

Check with your surgeon and doctor well in advance regarding which of your regular medications to continue or discontinue. On page 39 of this book, we discuss important recommendations, such as avoiding all aspirin and aspirin-containing products at least ten days before and after cosmetic surgery.

Do I continue to take my regular vitamins?

Many vitamins cause increased risk of bleeding and bruising. Please refer to our chart on page 40 for information regarding when to stop taking these before surgery. These include vitamin E, echinacea, garlic, ginger, ginseng, arnica, gingko biloba, and St. John's Wort.

What will I feel after the surgery?

Patients typically complain of a burning sensation, tenderness, or a sensation of having small paper cuts. These symptoms are not permanent and are generally alleviated with over-the-counter pain relievers.

Will I be able to drive myself home after my blepharoplasty procedure?

If sedation is used, then someone will need to drive you home after your surgery.

Will I need someone to help me out at home after my blepharoplasty procedure?

If possible, have someone to help you out for the first day or two after surgery. We usually ask patients to rest for a couple of days and to avoid strenuous activities.

When will my lids look normal after surgery?

Swelling and bruising will resolve after one to two weeks, but redness of the upper-lid incision may last several weeks. You may also feel small bumps under the upper incisions that can last for weeks. These are normal side effects of blepharoplasty and will resolve.

When are the stitches removed after blepharoplasty?
Stitches are removed on the sixth or seventh postoperative day. The removal will be painless as they are placed in a way that they simply slide out.

Are there visible scars after an eyelid lift?
The scars are hidden so that they are nearly invisible after a period of time. On the upper eyelids, the incision is placed on the natural eyelid crease, and this scar will fade. On the lower eyelids, the incision is hidden behind the eyelid or just under the eyelashes. The incisions, when placed well, will heal and be imperceptible.

When can I wear glasses?
Patients can wear glasses immediately after eyelid cosmetic surgery.

When can I wear contact lenses?
Contact lenses can be worn one week after upper-eyelid blepharoplasty and two weeks after lower-eyelid blepharoplasty.

When can I wear makeup?
You can wear makeup ten days after the surgery. About 70 percent of the swelling resolves in the first two weeks. The remainder takes about two months to fully resolve. However, this is mild swelling that is not perceptible.

When will I be able to return to work after my blepharoplasty procedure?
Patients are generally able to return to work about one week after the blepharoplasty procedure.

When can I exercise after my blepharoplasty procedure?
To achieve the best results of your blepharoplasty, it is important to give your body a chance to recuperate. You should stop your exercise regimen and avoid other strenuous activities for two to three weeks after your procedure. Start slowly and listen to your body as it will usually tell you when you may be overdoing it, with increased discomfort around the eyes.

What does blepharoplasty cost?

The total costs depend on whether you are correcting both sets of lids (upper *and* lower) or one set of lids (upper *or* lower). According to the American Society of Plastic Surgeons, the average cost of lower lid blepharoplasty with fat transfer is $5600, which includes operating room and anesthesia fees. A brow lift runs about $8600, which also includes operating room and anesthesia fees.

Our sliver procedure (upper lid only) runs about $2,300 when done in the office and an additional $1,300 if done in our surgical facility. The cost of an upper and lower blepharoplasty and fat transfers is approximately 7300 which includes the operating room and anesthesia fees.

Will my insurance pay for an eyelid lift?

In some cases an upper-eyelid lift may be covered by insurance if there is loose skin that significantly interferes with vision and daily activities. A visual-field examination (which measures peripheral vision) and standardized photographs can help you determine if your procedure will be covered. Lower-eyelid lifts are almost never covered by insurance as they are nearly always considered cosmetic.

Is it possible to get financing for a cosmetic procedure?

Financing is available for plastic-surgery procedures at almost all practices.

Is lower-blepharoplasty-revision surgery possible?

We do perform lower-eyelid-revision surgery. However, it is not recommended before at least one year has passed since the prior surgery. The best way to determine if revision surgery is right for you is to schedule an appointment with an experienced board-certified facial plastic surgeon for a detailed consultation specific to your needs.

Chapter 10

Before and After Blepharoplasty Photos

BRIGHTER, MORE RESTED, AND YOUNGER

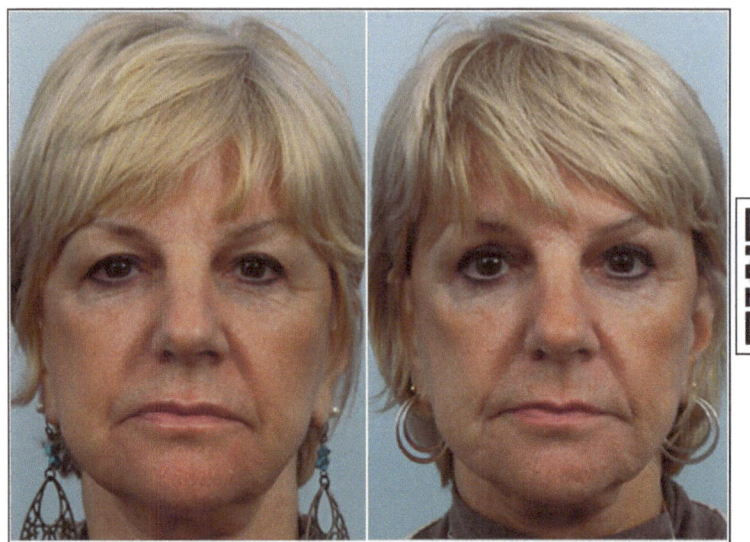

Scan for more information about this patient's upper eyelid surgery

Our Sliver Technique

This sixty-eight-year-old woman had a simple eyelid lift called a "sliver technique," which can be performed in an office setting. First, the upper eyelid is numbed with ice, and then a Novocain-type medication is injected so that patients feel little or no discomfort. A paper-cut-like incision is then made in the back crease of the eyelid, and then excess skin is removed, leaving the patient looking brighter, more rested, and younger as a result.

"I've always been conscious of no eyelids...my forehead has been seeping down over my eyes. The procedure (sliver technique) was easy...done right in the office, and it was like going to the dentist. I didn't feel anything, and it was done! I'd recommend the procedure in a minute!" - Scan code for video on this patient's experience of the sliver technique.

BLUE EYES SEEM BRIGHTER

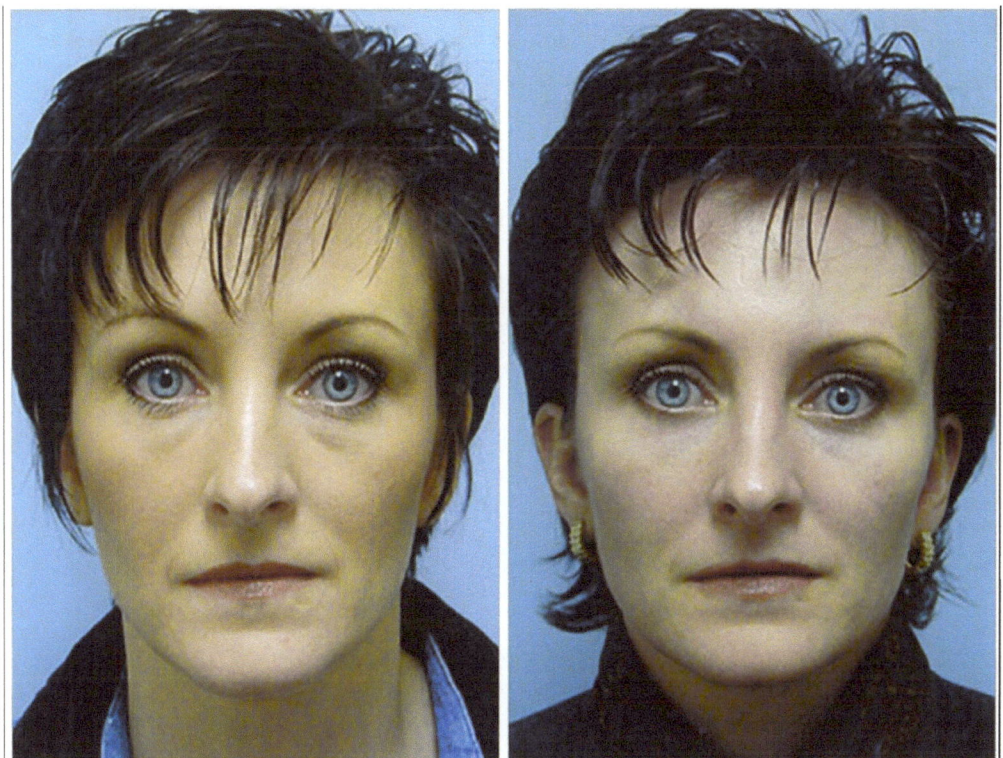 

Scan for more information about this patient's lower eye surgery

Lower-Eyelid Surgery

This patient, in her early thirties, complained of puffiness and wrinkling. A lower blepharoplasty was performed to remove eyelid fat as well as a TCA (trichloroacetic acid) chemical peel to tighten the skin. Her blue eyes seem brighter and more youthful as a result.

NO MORE BAGS

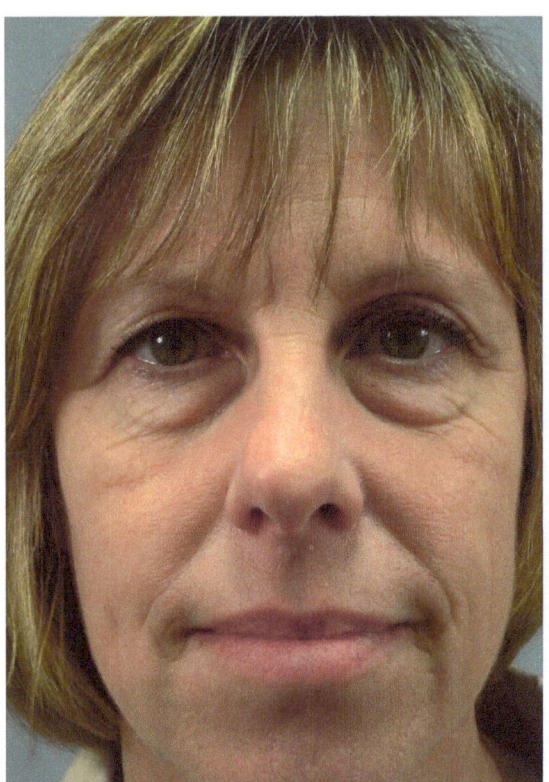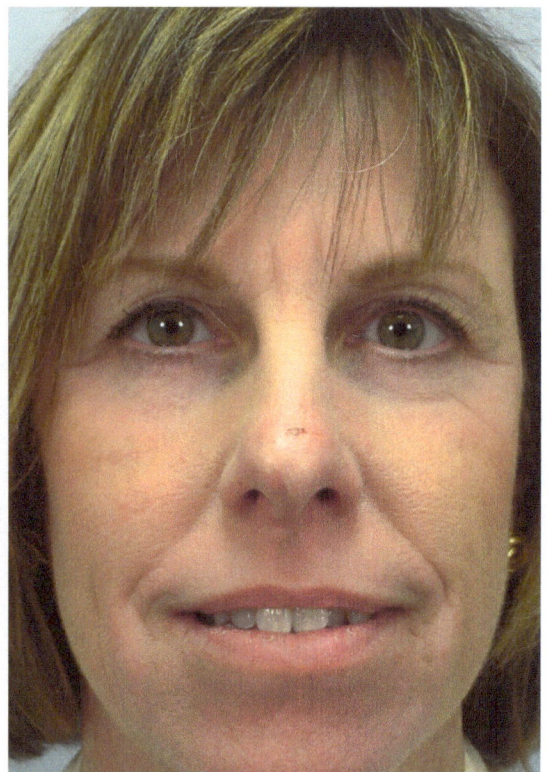

A Customized Surgical Approach

As you can see by her *before* picture, this woman has significant puffiness under her eyes. To correct this, a customized surgical approach was performed involving three different procedures: 1) a transcongentival incision (incision along the inside of the eyelid) to remove the fat pad causing the puffiness; 2) an incision just under the lower eyelashes to remove and tighten a small amount of skin; and 3) a chemical peel around the eyes and mouth to further smooth the skin.

A MORE RESTED LOOK

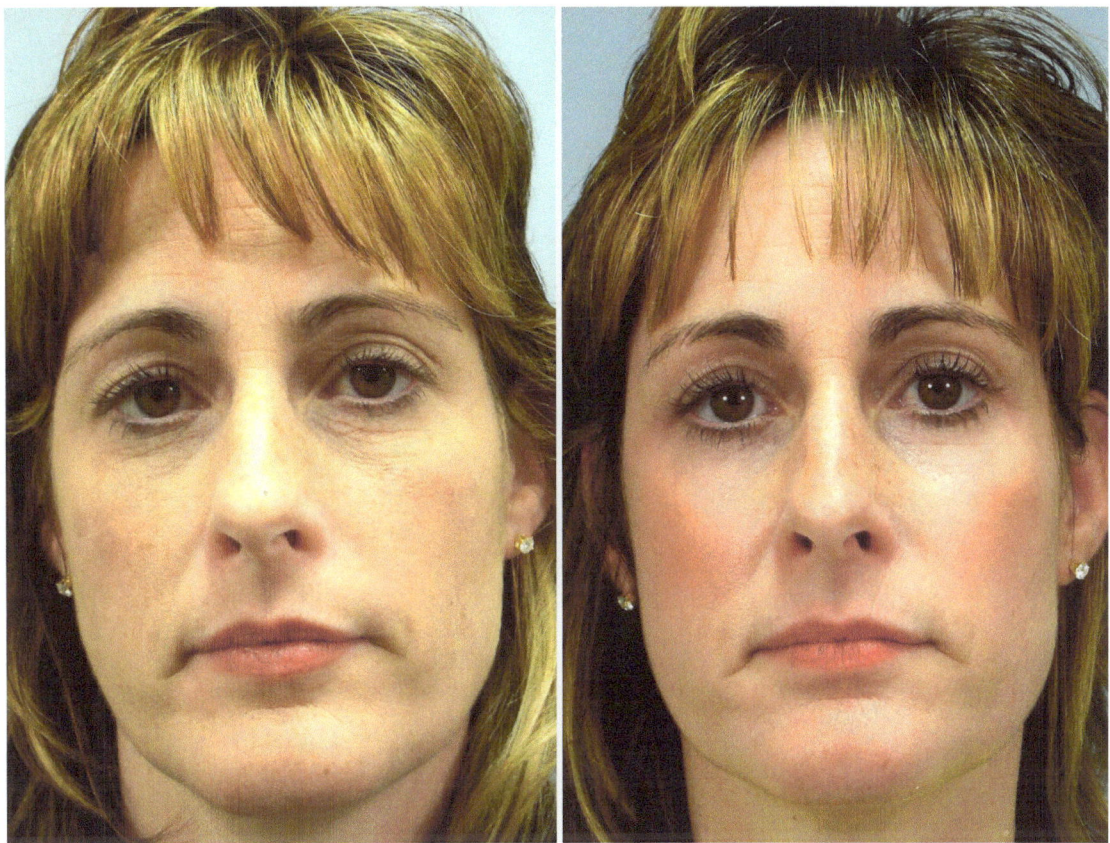

Sliver Technique and Chemical Peel

The patient, in her late thirties, had excess, loose skin on the upper eyelids, leaving her looking tired. After an upper blepharoplasty (our sliver technique) and a full-face chemical peel to diminish wrinkling on the lower lid, her eyes appear brighter, more rested, and refreshed.

YOUTHFUL AND MORE ATTRACTIVE

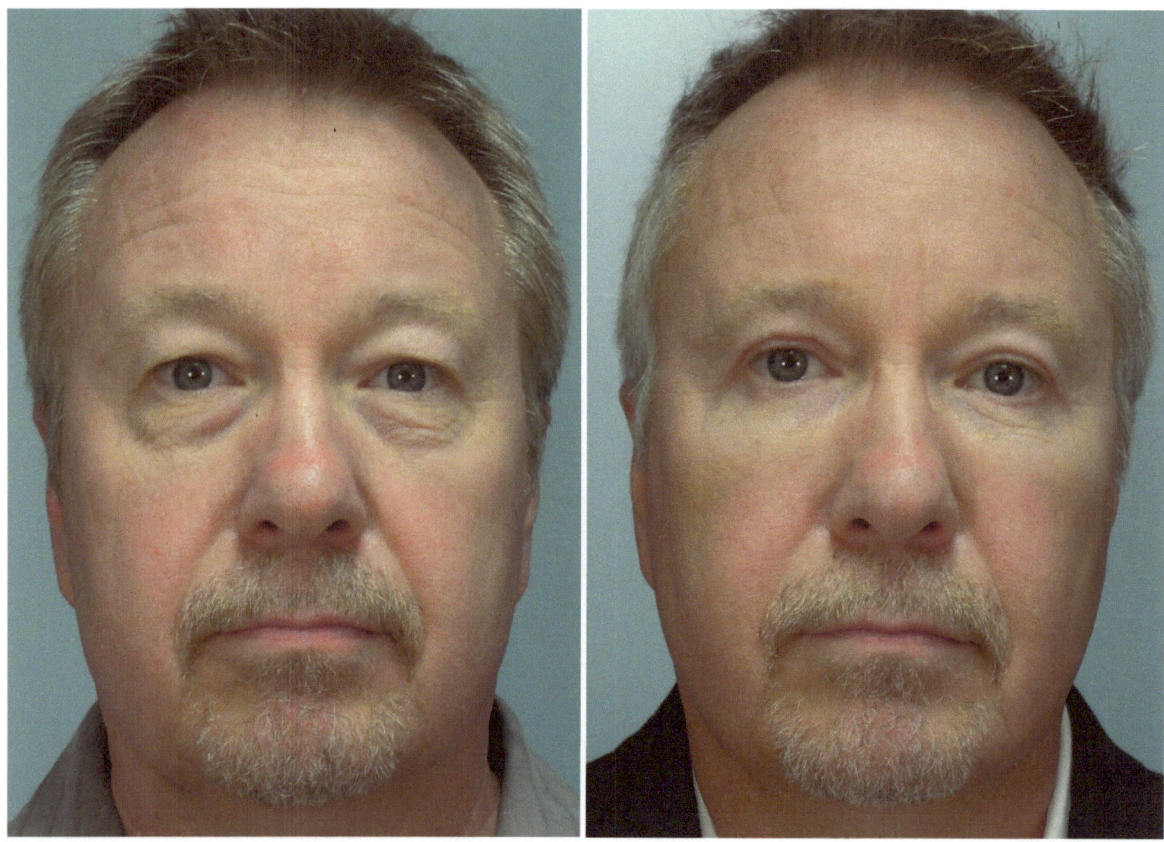

Lower-Lid Blepharoplasty

Aging around the eyes made this man look very tired and older than his forty-plus years. To correct the skin redundancy, wrinkles, and protruding under-eye fat, a lower-eyelid blepharoplasty as well as a fat transfer and removal of excess skin were performed. In the *after* photo taken six months later, he is looking considerably more rested and youthful. Notice there is no real change in the overall shape of his eyes, which is often very important to patients—just more of them are visible.

NO MORE PUFFINESS

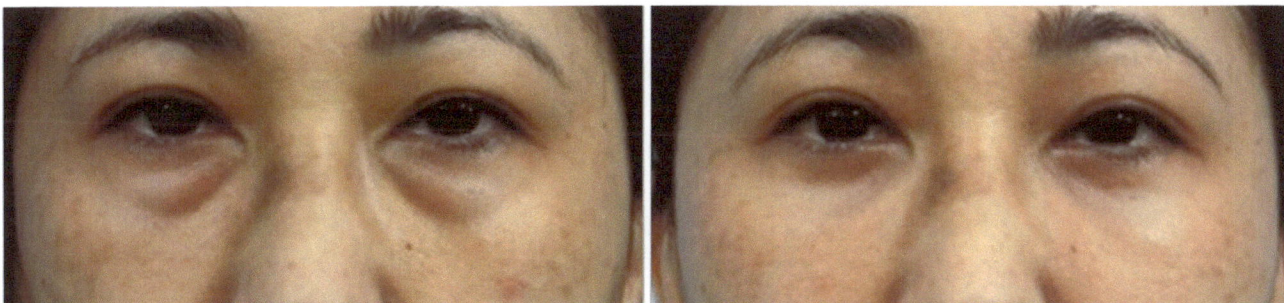

Fat Removed

This patient had protruding fat under her eyes that was removed through a tiny, invisible (transcongential) incision inside her eyelids. Then fat from her stomach was transferred to the hollow area under her eyes and throughout her midface. This is an example of a customized procedure where skin is not always removed.

HOLLOW-LOOKING EYES

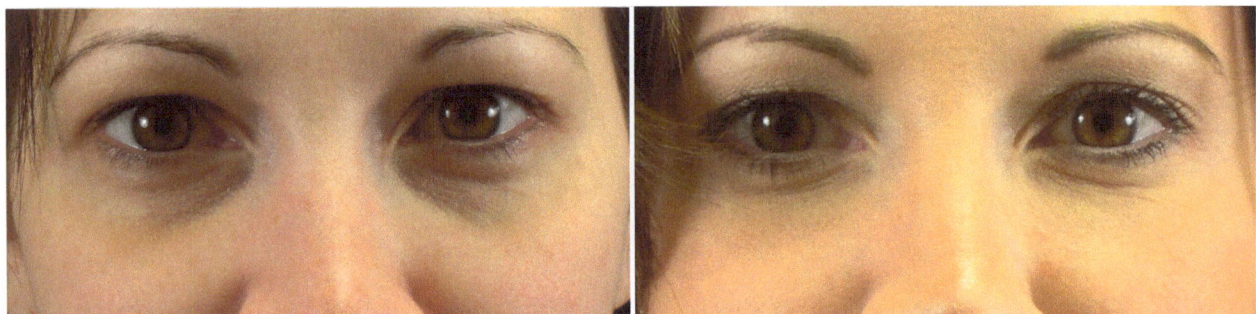

Nonsurgical Approach

Often a patient's genetic makeup is the cause of hollowing under the eye. However, other causes include normal aging and too much fat removed during a blepharoplasty. This patient, in her midthirties, chose a nonsurgical approach, using Restylane filler to address the hollowness as well as Botox injections to lift the brow. The result is a younger-looking face with no downtime, and results were visible in a matter of days.

MORE REFRESHED AND YOUTHFUL

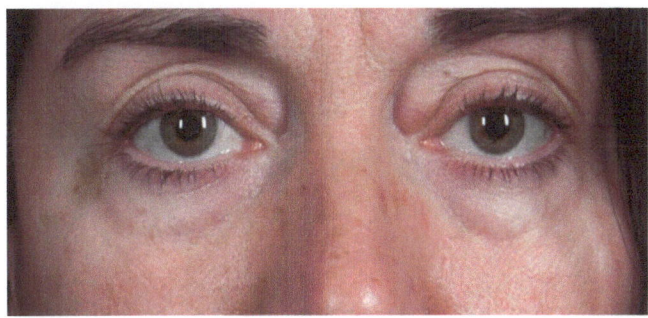 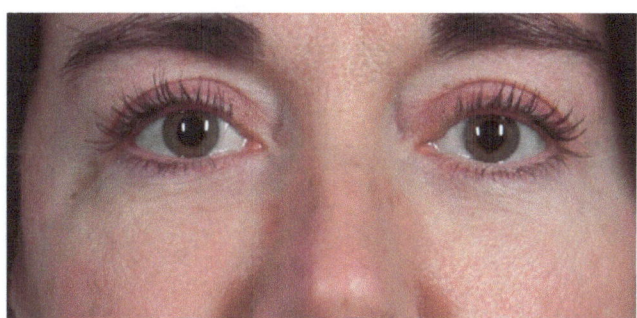

Sliver Technique and Lower-Lid Blepharoplasty

An incision (our sliver technique) was made in the crease of the upper eyelid, and excess skin and fat was removed from the corners of the lids. This creates more of a crease in the upper eyelid, resulting in less puffiness and a more youthful appearance.

This patient also had a lower-lid blepharoplasty and fat transfer to the midface to address the puffiness and hollowing *under* her eyes. Here, a tiny incision is made on the inside of the eyelid to remove the fat causing the puffiness. Fat from the abdominal area is used to fill in the hollow area under her eyes *and* along her upper eyelids.

This is an example of how we customize our patients' treatment to meet their specific concerns.

LESS PUFFINESS AND MORE DEFINITION

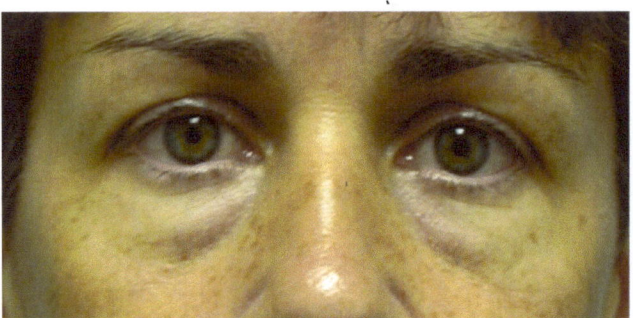 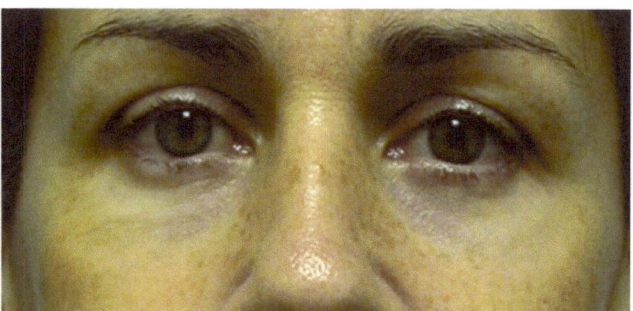

Lower-Lid Blepharoplasty and Chemical Peel

This patient complained of looking tired even when well-rested. A lower-lid blepharoplasty and a chemical peel to help tighten the lower-eyelid skin were performed, resulting a livelier and more refreshed look.

We typically recommend adding volume to the lower midface to create greater definition in the cheek and lower-lid areas. While this patient's appearance is improved, her outcome would have been enhanced by such a procedure.

ENVIRONMENT TAKES ITS TOLL

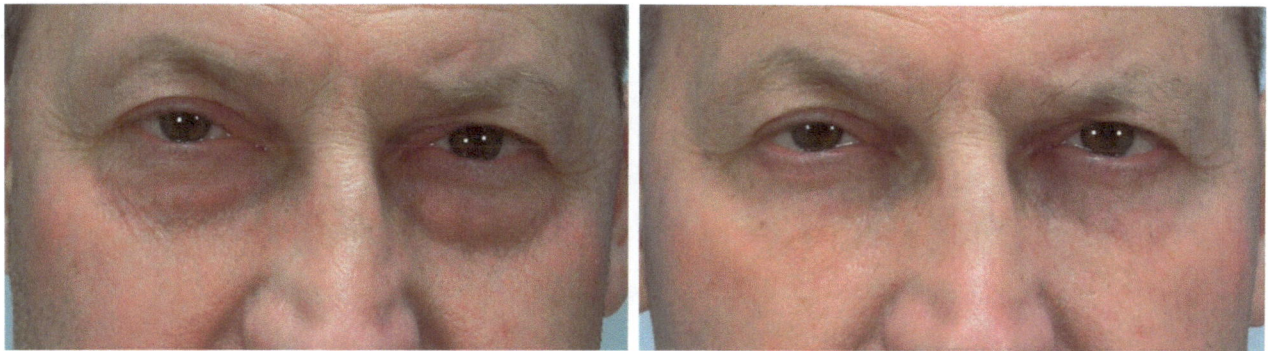

Lower-Eyelid Blepharoplasty and Fat Transfer

This military man in his early sixties spent a considerable amount of time overseas in a very hot and dusty climate, which may have contributed to a prematurely aged appearance. A lower-eyelid blepharoplasty was performed, removing the puffiness with an incision behind the eyelid and a fat transfer as well. You might notice a greater correction was needed on the left side of his face, which is common as one side of the face typically ages more than the other. His appearance looks more youthful and healthier.

RESTED, REFRESHED, REVIVED

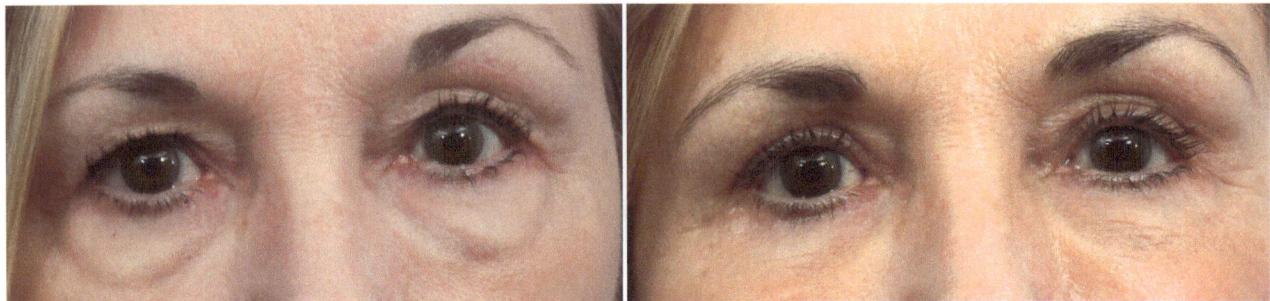

Lower-Lid Blepharoplasty and Fat Transfer

A lower-lid blepharoplasty removed the saggy, puffy skin under this patient's eyes. Fat was then transferred from her inner thighs and placed under her eyes and to the midface. She now looks more rested with a more defined cheek line, and her nasal folds appear softer as a result.

MAKEUP GOES ON SMOOTHER

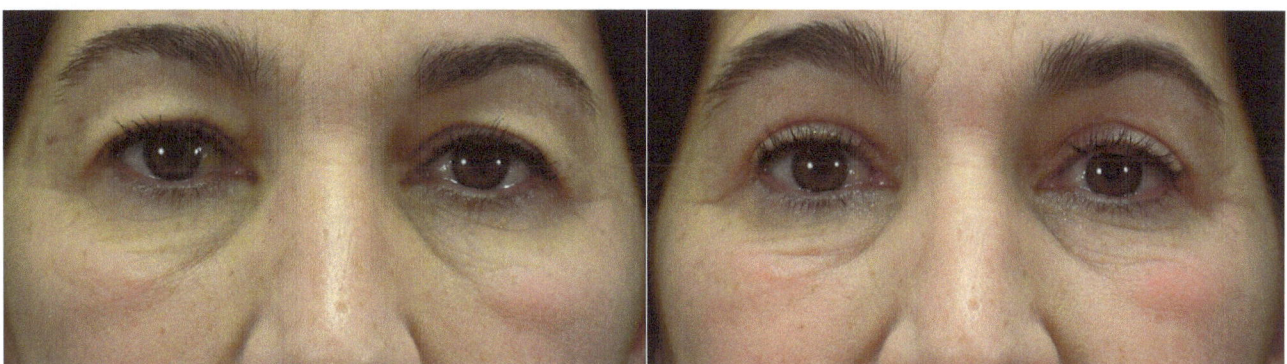

Sliver Technique

Excess skin on the upper eyelids can make it difficult to apply or wear eye makeup. Our sliver technique, a small paper-cut-like incision in the crease of the upper eyelid, performed in our office, removed the excess skin.

WELL-RESTED AND ALERT

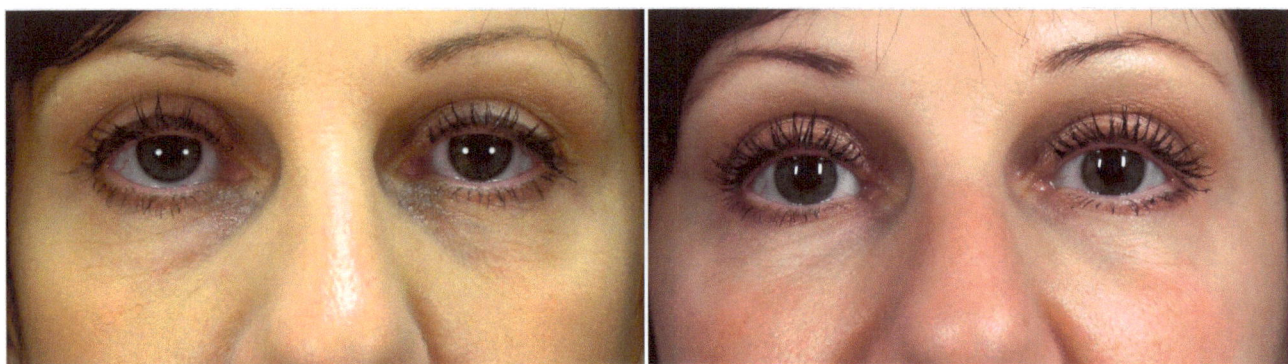

Nonsurgical Approach

Volume replacement with Restylane is one nonsurgical way to improve the appearance of lower eyelids with volume loss as shown in this patient's photos.

Restylane filler was placed in the tear trough (hollow area from corner of lower eyelid down) and along the orbital rim, which softened the hollowed area under her eyes, leaving this patient with a more rested look.

IMPROVED VISION AND VIBRANCY

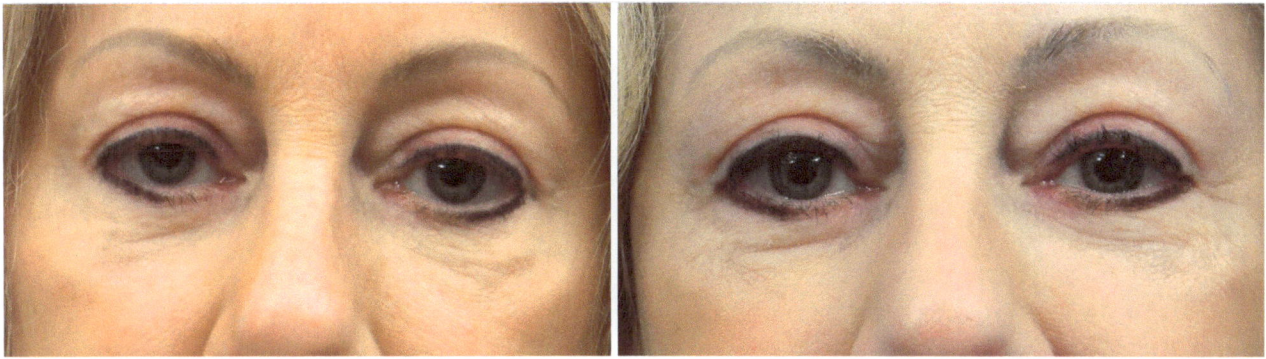

Ptosis Repair

This patient had ptosis repair to improve her vision. Ptosis is a condition where the upper eyelids hang over the pupils (black part of the eye). During surgery the muscle was adjusted so her upper lids are now resting at the level of the iris (colored part of the eye). This procedure also offers a more youthful, vibrant appearance.

TIRED OF LOOKING TIRED

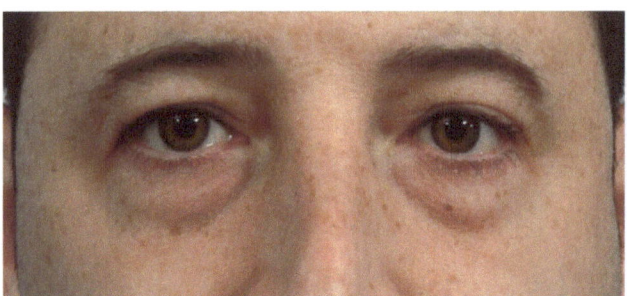 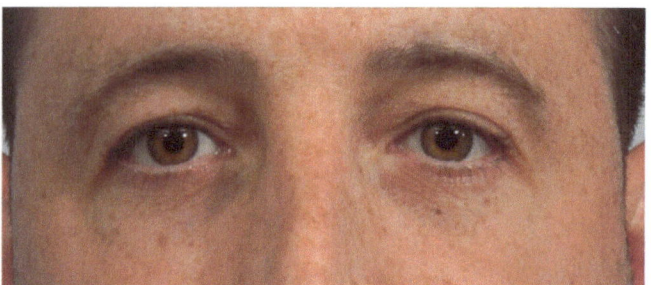

Lower-Lid Blepharoplasty and Fat Transfer

This thirty-seven-year-old man wanted to get rid of the bags under his eyes. The puffy fat and excess skin was removed. Fat was then transferred from his abdomen to the lower lid and midface. His result is a younger-looking and more energetic appearance.

About the Author

D
r. Edwin Williams is certified by the American Board of Facial Plastic and Reconstructive Surgery and the American Board of Otolaryngology and is a fellow of the American College of Surgeons. He serves as president of the Academy for Facial Plastic and Reconstructive Surgeons (2015–2016). He is also a diplomat of the National Board of Medical Examiners, a member of Alpha Omega Alpha Medical Honor Society, a fellow of the American Academy of Facial Plastic and Reconstructive Surgery and the American Academy of Otolaryngology—Head and Neck Surgery. With his active involvement in continuing medical education, Dr. Williams has qualified for the American Medical Association Physician Recognition Award.

Dr. Williams attended Cornell University in Ithaca, New York, where he received a bachelor of science in 1982. He began medical school at the State University of Buffalo School of Medicine and received his doctor of medicine in 1986. From 1986 to 1987, Dr. Williams completed his graduate internship in surgery at SUNY Health Sciences Center in Syracuse, New York.

Following this, he completed his residency training in otolaryngology—head and neck from 1987 to 1991. During his head and neck surgical training in Syracuse, Dr. Williams developed a strong interest in plastic surgery of the face, head, and neck. With a further desire for training in this area, he pursued a fellowship through the American Academy of Facial and Plastic Reconstructing Surgery at the University of Illinois in Chicago from 1991 to 1992. During this year of training, his entire experience consisted of cosmetic and reconstruction surgery of the nose, eyes, face, and neck.

Upon returning to the Northeast and beginning his practice in Albany, New York, Dr. Williams has continued to be actively involved in teaching facial plastic and reconstruction surgery to the residents of the Albany Medical Center and as former chief of the section of Facial and Plastic Reconstruction Surgery at Albany Medical Center, where he recently received an academic appointment of clinical professor in the Department of Surgery.

With an active involvement in lecturing and medical education, he continues to make presentations to various medical associations and has had numerous articles and chapters published in various major journals and textbooks.

www.ingramcontent.com/pod-product-compliance
Lightning Source LLC
Chambersburg PA
CBHW050731180526
45159CB00003B/1188